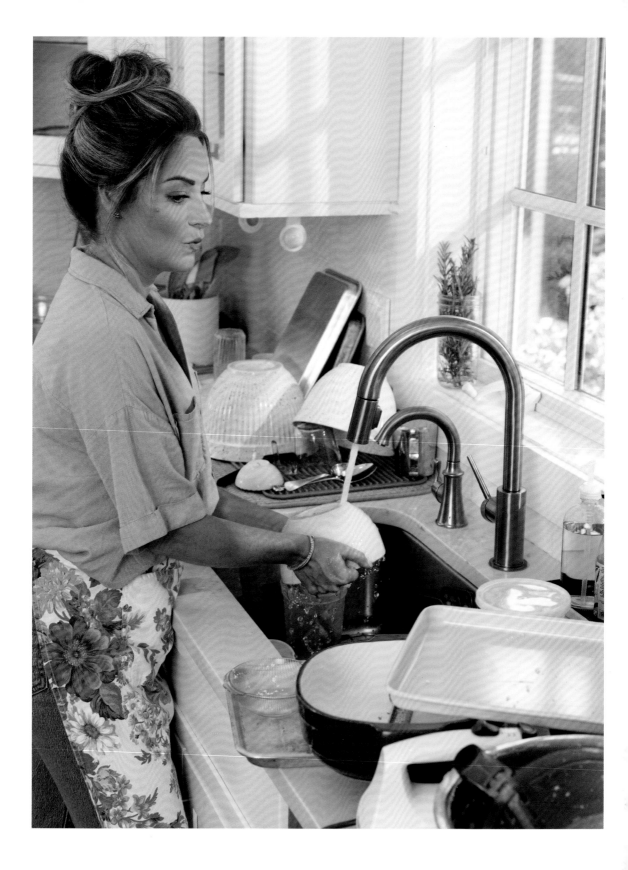

At the Kitchen Sink

RECIPES TO FILL YOUR TABLE,
WORDS TO FILL YOUR HEART

Dina Deleasa~Gonsar

CONVERGENT

New York

Published in the United States by Convergent Books, an imprint of Random House,
a division of Penguin Random House LLC, New York.

CONVERGENT with colophon is a registered trademark of Penguin Random House LLC.

Photographs in the collages on pages 224–225 and pages 246–248 are all courtesy of the
author, except for the group photo (left, middle row) on page 225 which is by Lauren Listor,
copyright © 2025 by Lauren Listor.

Library of Congress Cataloging-in-Publication Data
Names: Deleasa-Gonsar, Dina, author.
Title: At the kitchen sink / by Dina Deleasa-Gonsar.
Description: First edition. | New York, NY : Convergent, [2025] | Includes index.
Identifiers: LCCN 2024019976 (print) | LCCN 2024019977 (ebook) |
ISBN 9780593728932 (hardcover) | ISBN 9780593728949 (ebook)
Subjects: LCSH: Cooking. | Devotion. | LCGFT: Cookbooks.
Classification: LCC TX714 .D442 2025 (print) |
LCC TX714 (ebook) | DDC 641.5—dc23/eng/20240517
LC record available at https://lccn.loc.gov/2024019976
LC ebook record available at https://lccn.loc.gov/2024019977

Printed in China

convergentbooks.com

9 8 7 6 5 4 3 2 1

First Edition

Book design by Debbie Glasserman

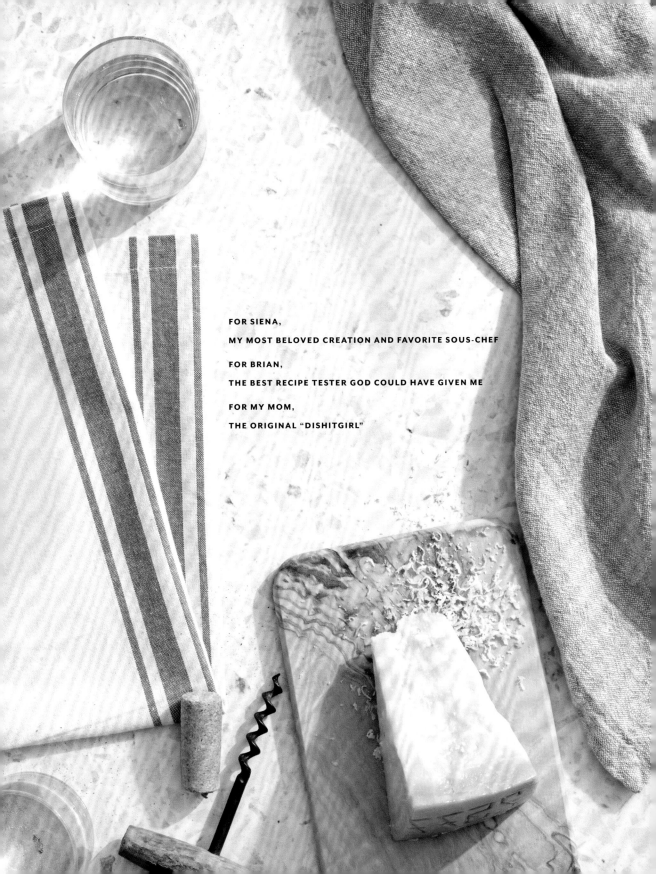

FOR SIENA,
MY MOST BELOVED CREATION AND FAVORITE SOUS-CHEF

FOR BRIAN,
THE BEST RECIPE TESTER GOD COULD HAVE GIVEN ME

FOR MY MOM,
THE ORIGINAL "DISHITGIRL"

Contents

At the Kitchen Sink

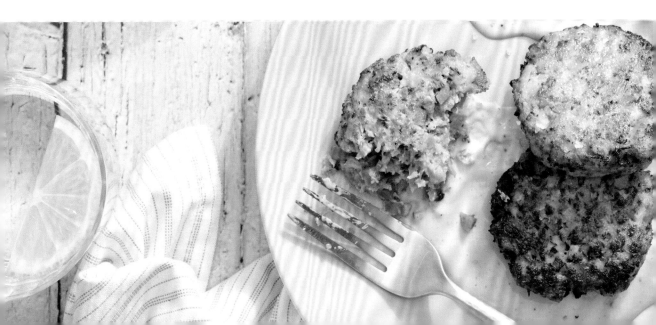

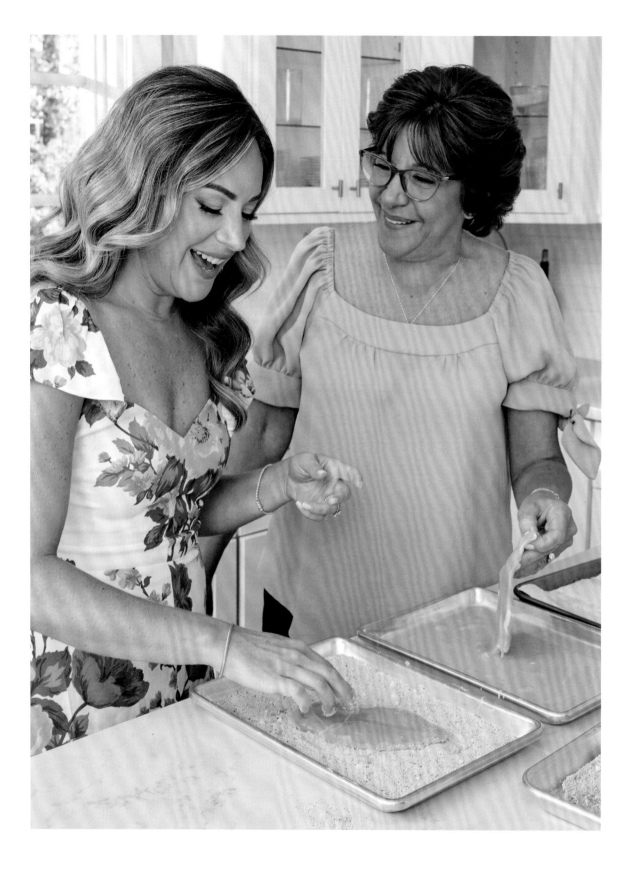

Introduction

Have you ever stood over the kitchen sink and asked God to help you make it through the day? The water is running, and you take a deep breath, gripping the counter in front of you as you summon the strength to make it to bedtime. Maybe you're hiding tears from the ones you love the most because you do not want to worry them. Or maybe you're washing baby bottles, delirious from two months of almost no sleep, wondering what happened to your life.

But then these moments give way to the countless times when you're in the opposite scenario. You're over the kitchen sink loading the dishwasher after a busy Sunday dinner. Your children's cousins, dressed up in princess outfits, are running around the kitchen island. Your dad sits on the couch laughing at them while your mother and sister carry on a lively conversation in the dining room. You smile to yourself and think about how a moment such as this, in your home, is what you prayed for: a home full of a lovable chaos, with you and your family carrying on family traditions and building a life full of memories, much as your parents did.

In both of these scenarios, I have stood at the kitchen sink and learned that each tear shed brings us that much closer to our next triumph. God hasn't promised us a journey without valleys, but we can let him carry us through the hard moments of life, rejoicing with him through the wilderness as well as in the promised land.

It isn't always easy, but it is always purposeful. God has entrusted the people in your care to you specifically. He has called you to such a time as this, and I am confident that he will equip you and give you a strength you didn't know you could have.

This is a cookbook, with inspiration and a helping hand, for each part of that journey—no matter what your kitchen sink looks like. Many of the recipes come from my childhood, growing up in a large Italian American family that gathered every week for Sunday dinners. When my grandmother passed away, her jewelry or knickknacks didn't interest me. Instead, I asked for her apron, saved a piece of vintage Pyrex from the discard pile, and begged for her handwritten recipes, not only because I wanted to cook from them but because I knew she'd held the pen to form the words. When I'm cooking, her kitchen is the one I go back to in the corners of my mind, and many of the recipes in this book are ones she and my mother served for years.

Life is different than it was back then. As a working mom who's raising a family and navigating a schedule full of extracurricular activities, I have switched up my kitchen philosophy, making room for recipes that allow for the kitchen table to transfer to the back seat of an SUV and repurposing a rotisserie chicken in ways that make me feel like a genius. Whether you're scraping by on a busy weeknight, planning a big meal for a celebratory gathering, or reminding yourself to eat in the middle of a busy afternoon, my hope is to help you nourish your family and community—and your spirit along the way.

Each chapter also contains devotions to remind you of God's presence. I want to do so much more than build your cooking skills—I want to support you in your everyday life and work. I want to remind you that God sees your heart and your obedience and that your faithful efforts do not go unnoticed in his kingdom. Read these devotions in a season when your kitchen sink is the quietest place in your house and when you're drowning in the monotony of the mundane.

Overall, this book aims to become not just another cookbook on your shelf but a part of your family. Like a photo album on the coffee table, I hope it will inspire you to create traditions and family rhythms. Those who are no longer here are never truly gone. The home we foster and the faith that sustains us will become the legacy we leave behind, and that legacy will keep our families coming back to the table for years to come. God has entrusted your family to you for a divine reason. He sees your faithfulness; it does not go unnoticed. There is something marvelous in your mundane, and there is purpose in your prayers at the kitchen sink.

This book is a love letter to my family. Let me encourage you to begin writing yours.

Getting Started

Pantry Picks

We all have a certain few spices and ingredients that are constants in our kitchens, but the beauty of trying new recipes is that it introduces us to new flavors, textures, and ingredients. For example, you may have never considered adding cardamom to banana bread (page 197). However, soon you will be adding it to dishes just as much as you now add cinnamon. Or you'll try the Smoky Sweet Potato and Farro Bowl (page 107), and before you know it, smoked paprika becomes an even more common ingredient you use than plain paprika.

Just one simple spice swap can change up your everyday routine. It's also another way to learn about other countries and cultures.

Keeping budget in mind, I suggest purchasing one new item per grocery trip. Keep your eyes peeled for a sale on a fun new vinegar or oil, and try a smaller bottle at first as opposed to the larger sizes. Stocking your kitchen with basics means you can focus more on the perimeter of the store when you grocery shop. It also increases variety in your meals and encourages spur-of-the-moment creativity.

The pantry items that follow have become constants in my kitchen. While some ingredients such as garlic powder or olive oil were adopted from my family's frequent use of them, others came about as I tried new recipes or experienced new flavors when traveling. For example, Chinese five spice was not something I had seen in my mother's kitchen, but I adopted it as a staple after using it in stir-fry recipes. From there, it made its way into other dishes, like the Saucy Baby Back Ribs (page 186). Now I couldn't imagine making the dry rub without it!

I find that many of the following ingredients elevate simple dishes in unexpected ways. For example, many people fear anchovies, but melted into tomato sauce, they give it a deep umami saltiness that couldn't be more different from the fishy taste people expect. Mascarpone cheese can make baked ziti feel very luxurious and also give the creamiest texture to desserts.

Follow your intuition, and feel free to swap ingredients according to your taste. You may prefer dried cranberries to dried cherries in salads or grain bowls. Or maybe Kalamata olives aren't your thing, but you love green olives. It's your kitchen. Experimenting with ingredient swaps is how you find your new favorites! However, it should be noted that not all salts are created equal. Diamond Crystal kosher salt is what I have in my kitchen and what was used to test the recipes. It is important to note that different brands of kosher salt could yield different results, and it's always important to taste your dishes throughout the cooking process to help you season them to your liking.

OILS AND VINEGARS

Coconut oil
Extra-virgin olive oil
Apple cider vinegar
Red wine vinegar
Balsamic vinegar
Balsamic glaze

SPICES AND DRIED HERBS

Kosher salt
Celery salt
Onion powder
Garlic powder
Dried basil
Dried thyme
Dried rosemary
Dried parsley
Crushed red pepper flakes
Smoked paprika
Ground cardamom
Chinese five spice
Ground mustard
Ground cumin
Black peppercorns
Bay leaves

CANS AND JARS

Yellowfin tuna in olive oil
Pitted Kalamata olives
Capers
Chickpeas
Pureed pumpkin
Marinated artichokes
Anchovy fillets

GRAINS AND STARCHES

Dried pasta (my favorites are bucatini, rigatoni, and penne)
Farro
Pearl couscous
Long grain white rice
Italian-style bread crumbs
Panko bread crumbs

NUTS, SEEDS, AND BUTTERS

Cookie butter
Chocolate hazelnut spread
Walnuts
Pecans
Chia seeds

SWEETENERS

Pure maple syrup
Honey
Coconut sugar
Light and dark brown sugar

BAKING

All-purpose flour
Dried cherries
Golden raisins
Semisweet chocolate chips
Unsweetened coconut flakes
Coconut chips
Vanilla extract
Almond extract

FRIDGE

Pancetta
Large eggs

FREEZER

Frozen spinach
Frozen popcorn chicken
Pierogies

**PRESERVES AND
PICKLES**

Hot cherry peppers in brine
Sliced pepperoncini

**CONDIMENTS
AND SAUCES**

Low-sodium soy sauce
Anchovy paste
Chipotle sauce
Worcestershire sauce
Hot honey

PRODUCE

Lemons
Apples
Bananas
Yellow, red, and green
   bell peppers
Red leaf lettuce
Arugula
Purple cabbage
Broccoli
Green beans
Cherry or grape tomatoes
Russet potatoes

Carrots
Avocados
Garlic
Shallots
Red onions
Yellow onions

DAIRY

Unsalted butter
Cream cheese
Whole milk ricotta cheese
Mascarpone cheese
Heavy cream
Whole milk
Unsweetened almond milk
Parmigiano-Reggiano
   cheese
Gruyère cheese
Feta cheese
Shredded mozzarella
Burrata cheese

ALCOHOL

Dry sherry
Dry white wine
Dry red wine

More to Share

One of the things that makes me the happiest is being able to share food with others. This goes beyond getting my loved ones together for Sunday dinner. When a friend has a baby, I never show up without a lasagna. Through my church, I often volunteer to cook for someone who is sick or going through a challenging season. Even during my busiest weeks, dropping off a meal is always worth the extra mile. I include my daughter, Siena, in these deliveries, and she now looks forward to coming along and ringing the doorbell. It serves as quality time for the two of us, all while helping illustrate a helper's heart.

Throughout the book, you'll notice that some of the recipes are marked as a "More to Share" recipe. These are my go-to dishes when cooking for a friend or a neighbor. These recipes can also feed a larger crowd or provide more than just one meal. They "travel" well, and I've found that they appeal to a wide range of palates.

More to Share Recipes

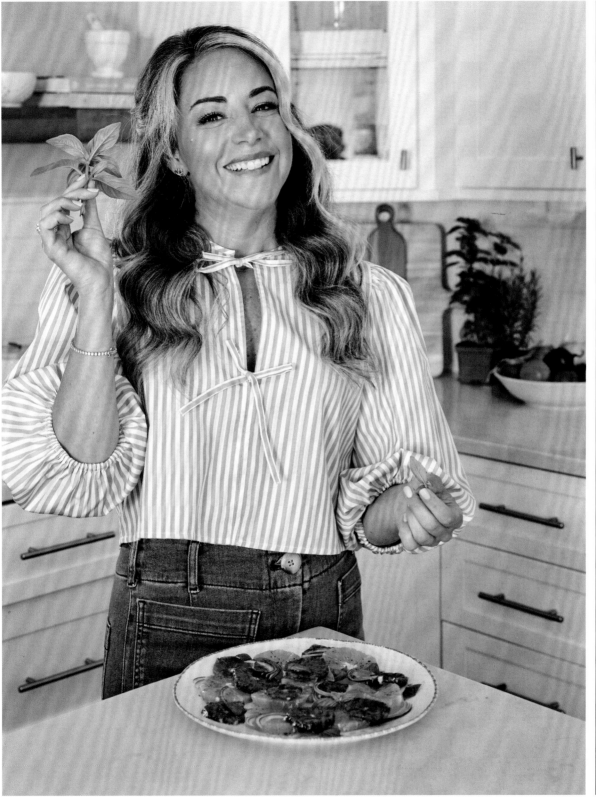

1
___
Morning Person:
Wake~Up Call

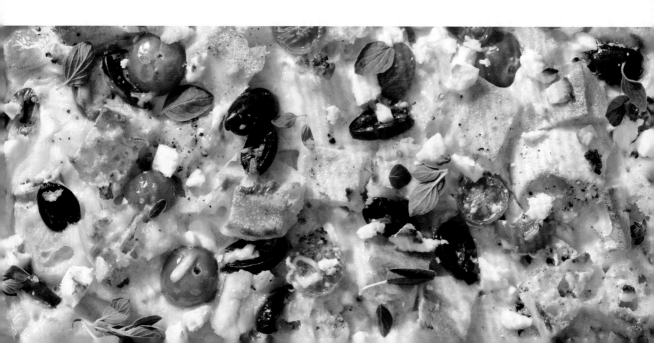

When we rise each day, we have a choice to make. We can start the day with dread, feeling anxious and overwhelmed, or we can tap into God's promises of peace and strength, allowing him to help reframe our day. We can lean in to his promise that his mercies are new every morning, trusting that he truly holds the future and has our best interest at heart.

There are so many blessings to experience when our eyes stay fixed on him. When we meditate on these things, rather than our anxieties, we can face the day refreshed and expectant, knowing he is there to carry us if need be.

Some mornings are made to be slow, when we can pour an extra cup of coffee and indulge in Carrot Cake Pancakes with Brown Sugar Cream Cheese Icing (page 22). Other mornings have us dashing out the door after grabbing a Lemon Coconut Oat Muffin (page 15). Regardless of which one you are experiencing, starting your day with filling your belly as well as your heart is a best practice.

Let the morning bring me word of your unfailing love,
   for I have put my trust in you.
Show me the way I should go,
   for to you I entrust my life.

PSALM 143:8

Quite a few verses in the Bible mention the morning. Usually it is referenced in a positive way. Lamentations 3 talks about the steadfast love of the Lord, reminding us that his mercies are new every day. Psalm 30 encourages us to hang in there and rejoice through hard times because joy comes in the morning. There is something about the start of a new day—a sense of possibility and the chance to start over again. Maybe that is why so many people suggest beginning your day with prayer or time in Scripture. There seems to be so much potential for productivity as we start our days. Why start without our hearts and minds fixed on God?

Well, maybe you were up late the night before, tossing and turning. Or your children love the sunrise just as much as you love the sunset. Maybe you pressed the snooze button on the alarm clock one too many times and now you're haphazardly putting waffles in the toaster oven and packing lunch. Most mornings aren't as romantic as people make them out to be on their morning routine reels.

While you may not be able to light a scented candle and read your Bible in the wee hours of the morning, that doesn't mean God can't do a new thing in your life. Don't get me wrong. There are some mornings where I do manage fifteen extra minutes for prayer before the rest of the house wakes up. But instead of beating myself up on the days when I can't do that, I find another way. Maybe I take a minute to pray after Siena leaves for school, or I read a verse from the list I keep in my prayer journal before I hop on the first Zoom call of the day.

I want God to know I am seeking him each and every day, first thing. I will no doubt encounter challenges throughout the day. There are many days when I must pray my way through the waves of emotions and anxiety that threaten to overtake me. Starting my morning with prayer is a way to make sure one challenging day doesn't overshadow the next. My prayer most days is, *Yesterday did not go as planned, but, Lord, I place today in your hands*.

> In the morning, LORD, you hear my voice;
>   in the morning I lay my requests before you
>   and wait expectantly.
>
> PSALM 5:3

The word *expectantly* rings in my ears. When we wait, confident in knowing that God will move, it changes everything. We begin the day with hope, mercy, and grace, instead of frustration, defeat, and confusion. Even if the rest of your morning is filled with rushed moments, lost shoes, or an email that threatens the trajectory of the day, God can still do a new thing. No matter how night threatens us, let's move forward with the promise of the morning.

———————————

Dear Lord, walk with me throughout the day. Help me know that you are near and that circumstances of yesterday do not have to dictate today. If I feel off balance, please set my feet upon the rock. Help me give myself grace in the moments I feel like I am failing, and remind me of your mercy and kindness. Fill my heart with hope and expectancy instead of dread and defeat.

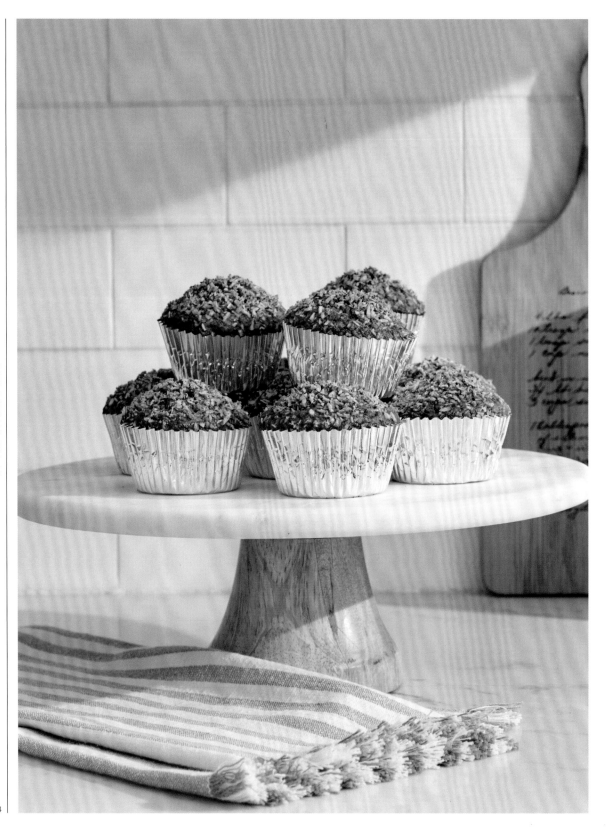

Lemon Coconut Oat Muffins

MAKES: 12 MUFFINS | PREP: 15 MINUTES | COOK: 20 MINUTES | INACTIVE: 15 MINUTES

My favorite thing about these muffins is the crunchy coconut topping. Coconut sugar has a more caramelized taste than granulated sugar. The subtle squeeze of lemon juice brightens up the batter, making the muffins a delightful morning treat!

1½ cups quick-cooking rolled oats

1 cup whole milk

1 cup all-purpose flour

½ cup plus 3 tablespoons unsweetened shredded coconut

1¼ teaspoons baking powder

½ teaspoon baking soda

1 teaspoon ground cinnamon

⅛ teaspoon kosher salt

2 large eggs, lightly beaten

¾ cup plus 2 tablespoons coconut sugar

⅓ cup vegetable oil

1 tablespoon freshly squeezed lemon juice

2 teaspoons lemon zest

1. Preheat the oven to 425°F. Line a standard 12-cup muffin pan with paper or aluminum foil liners.

2. In a large bowl, stir together the oats and milk until combined. Set aside to soften for 15 minutes.

3. In a medium bowl, whisk together the flour, ½ cup of the shredded coconut, the baking powder, baking soda, cinnamon, and salt.

4. Add the eggs, ¾ cup of the coconut sugar, the oil, lemon juice, and lemon zest to the soaked oats and mix well to combine. Add the dry ingredients and mix until well combined.

5. Divide the batter among the lined cavities, filling each almost to the top of the liners.

6. In a small bowl, stir together the remaining 3 tablespoons shredded coconut and remaining 2 tablespoons coconut sugar to combine. Sprinkle over the batter.

7. Bake for 5 minutes and then, without opening the oven, lower the temperature to 350°F and continue baking until a toothpick inserted into the center of a muffin comes out clean, about 15 minutes more.

8. Let the muffins cool in the pan for 10 minutes before removing. Serve warm or at room temperature.

MORE TO SHARE RECIPE

NOTE

You can substitute ½ cup of packed light brown sugar for the coconut sugar.

Nutella Crescent Roll Breakfast Bake

SERVES: 6 TO 8 | PREP: 15 MINUTES | COOK: 30 MINUTES

I am a big fan of make-ahead breakfasts, and this baked dish is great to have prepared as you head into the weekend. Nutella and strawberries make it feel more special than a weekday breakfast, but you can throw it in the oven when you wake up and it'll be ready right before you head out for a day on the go.

½ cup whole milk ricotta cheese

¼ cup Nutella or chocolate hazelnut spread of your choice

1¼ teaspoons ground cinnamon, divided

2 (8-ounce) cans crescent rolls

3 large eggs

3 tablespoons heavy cream

1 teaspoon vanilla extract

3 tablespoons unsalted butter, melted

1 tablespoon sugar

¾ cup chopped strawberries

1. Preheat the oven to 375°F. Coat a 9 by 13-inch baking dish with nonstick cooking spray.

2. In a medium bowl, whisk together the ricotta, Nutella, and ¼ teaspoon of the cinnamon until well combined.

3. Remove the crescent rolls from the cans, unroll the dough, and cut along the perforated lines to make triangles. Place about 1 teaspoon of the Nutella mixture along the long side of each triangle, smoothing it across the top with the back of a spoon. Roll each triangle into a crescent and place them in the prepared baking dish, making two rows of eight rolls.

4. In a medium bowl, whisk together the eggs, cream, and vanilla. Pour the mixture over the top of the rolls.

5. Bake for 15 minutes.

6. Meanwhile, in a small bowl, stir together the butter, sugar, and the remaining 1 teaspoon of cinnamon.

7. Using a pastry brush, carefully brush the butter mixture over the partially baked rolls.

8. Return to the oven and bake until the tops are golden brown and the rolls are set in the middle, about 15 minutes more. Cool for 5 to 10 minutes, then sprinkle the strawberries over the top and serve warm.

NOTE

The recipe, up to the baking, can be made the night before.

Leftovers can be heated in the toaster oven or microwave.

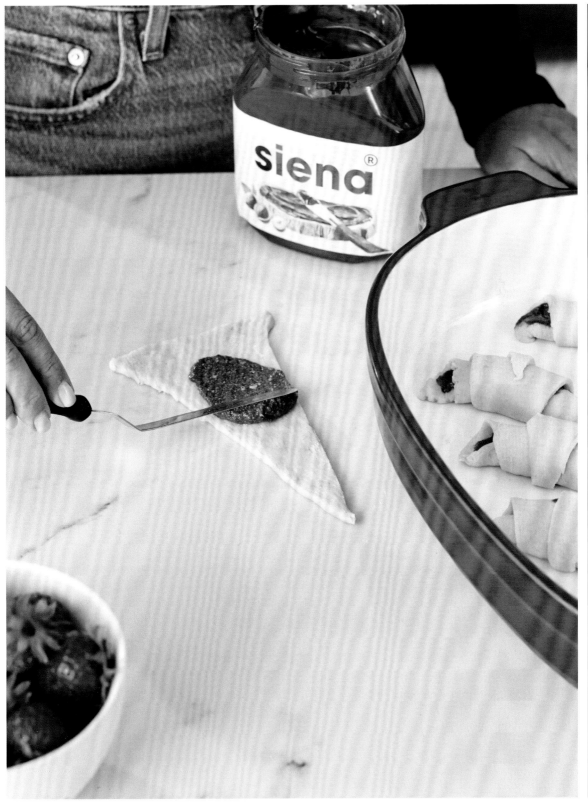

Have you ever gone through a time when you were just *killing* it? You were waking up every day, drinking water first thing, getting a workout in, being mindful of what you ate, and those habits left you feeling more energized and motivated as you effortlessly checked off your to-do list. You never wanted to fall out of this routine. Then came the morning when you woke up late or one of the kids caught the stomach flu. You missed a workout and started drinking more coffee than you should. One day of being off schedule turned into one week, and soon you not only were off track but also had no willpower to return.

Most of us have been caught in this cycle more than we care to admit. We tell ourselves that it will always be too hard for us to start over again and that we will always fall short, so why even bother?

As I waded through postpartum depression, I often struggled with these thoughts. I felt as if Siena was always crying and unhappy. It seemed like every time I would take her to the park or on an outing, she was fussy. Or I would plan to do the laundry and prep dinner during her nap, but that nap would never happen. I started staring out the kitchen sink window, resigning within myself that it would always be like this.

When our days are overwhelming, we look for somewhere to place the blame. We start dwelling on the disappointing or challenging circumstances in front of us, and they take on a sort of permanency in our daily routine. This thought pattern becomes familiar and comfortable. We can get so deep in this cycle that even when circumstances change, we fail to recognize it because we are stuck. We forget that God's mercies are new every morning and that we do not have to subscribe to the finality of our problems. This is where Satan wants us to be. He wants us to be like Israelites, wandering in the desert for forty years, forgetting about the manna and all the victories and deliverance God has offered along the way.

But You, O Lord, be merciful and gracious to me, and raise me
up, that I may requite them.
By this I know that You favor and delight in me, because my
enemy does not triumph over me.
And as for me, You have upheld me in my integrity and set me in
Your presence forever.

PSALM 41:10–12, AMPC

Let's not be all-or-nothing in how we face our days but instead tap into the grace that God gives. Things might be slow, but thank God you are making small steps in waking up to face each day. Today, the baby may be fussy, your list of chores may go unchecked, and dinner might never happen, but tomorrow is a new day. And even if it feels as though you are making no progress or your business is stalling or your résumé is going unread, God is working where you cannot see. There is always a chance for restoration, reconciliation, and renewal. The devil would have you believe your circumstances are insurmountable, that the prison of your negative thoughts and emotions is where you belong. But Jesus says, "Bring them to me and let's begin again."

Dear Lord, fix my eyes on you today. Help me tune in to your words of encouragement, forsaking discouragement. Help me temper my emotions, knowing that this valley isn't forever. My problems do not have the final say. You do.

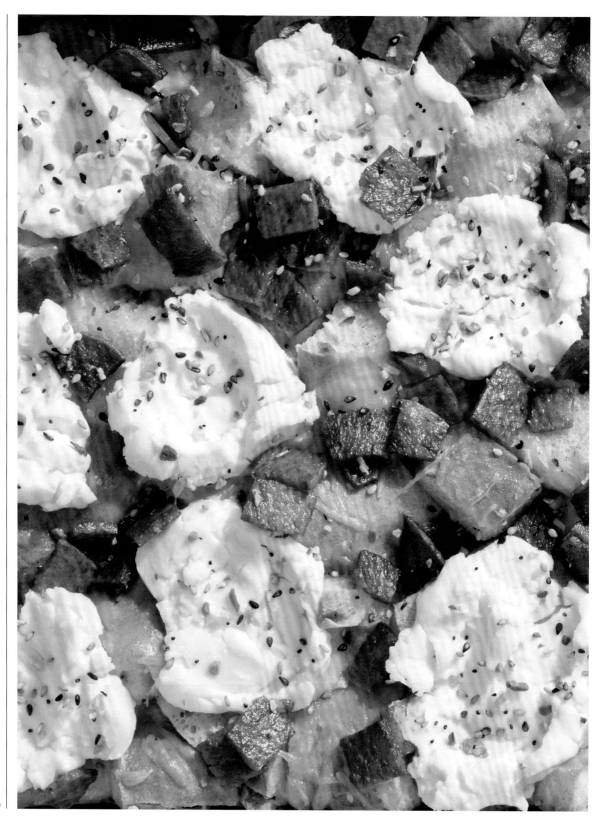

Jersey Bagel Egg Strata

SERVES: 8 | PREP: 15 MINUTES | COOK: 1 HOUR | INACTIVE: 6 HOURS

There is nothing better than Taylor ham, egg, and cheese on a New Jersey–made bagel. Or maybe you know it as a pork roll, egg, and cheese. This debate is as heated as asking two Italian Americans if their meatballs are in gravy or sauce on Sunday! No matter what you call it, this breakfast casserole will always hit close to home!

8 slices of Taylor ham (or pork roll)

10 large eggs

2 cups whole milk

2 tablespoons everything bagel seasoning

1 teaspoon kosher salt

½ teaspoon ground black pepper

4 large plain bagels, cut in 1-inch cubes (about 6 cups)

1½ cups shredded Cheddar cheese

1 (8-ounce) package cream cheese, softened

1. Heat a large skillet over medium heat. Add the Taylor ham in batches, and cook, turning once, until the edges are crisped, about 2 minutes per side. Transfer to a plate to cool, then cut into bite-size pieces.

2. Meanwhile, in a large bowl, whisk together the eggs, milk, bagel seasoning, salt, and pepper until well combined.

3. Spread the bagel cubes evenly in a 9 by 13-inch baking dish. Pour the egg mixture over the top, gently pressing the bagel cubes to make sure they're coated with the egg mixture. Sprinkle the Cheddar cheese evenly over the top, then add dollops of cream cheese, about 1 tablespoon each, followed by the ham. Cover with plastic wrap and refrigerate for at least 6 hours, preferably overnight.

4. Preheat the oven to 375°F.

5. Bake, uncovered, about 35 minutes.

6. Remove from the oven and use the back of a spoon to carefully spread the cream cheese over the top of the casserole.

7. Return to the oven and continue baking until the center is set and the edges begin to brown, about 15 minutes more. Let sit for 5 minutes before serving.

NOTE

If you want this to be true "Jersey" style, serve with a squeeze of ketchup! Unless you are like my husband Brian, who is from Pennsylvania and despises ketchup.

Carrot Cake Pancakes
with Brown Sugar Cream Cheese Icing

MAKES: 10 PANCAKES | PREP: 20 MINUTES | COOK: 15 MINUTES | INACTIVE: 30 MINUTES

A couple of years ago, I won Hallmark Channel's Best Home Cook on its *Home & Family* show—one of the highlights of my career. After the contest, I was lucky enough to join them periodically for cooking segments throughout the next year. In one of my first episodes with them, I made these pancakes. They are perfect for a springtime brunch or Easter Sunday. The brown sugar and cream cheese icing make these pancakes a real treat!

FOR THE PANCAKES

3 medium carrots, peeled

1½ cups all-purpose flour

¼ cup granulated sugar

1 tablespoon light or dark brown sugar

1 teaspoon baking powder

¼ teaspoon baking soda

½ teaspoon fine sea salt

½ teaspoon ground cinnamon

¼ teaspoon ground ginger

¼ teaspoon ground nutmeg

1 cup whole milk

2 large eggs

1 teaspoon vanilla extract

2 tablespoons unsalted butter

2 tablespoons golden raisins, or
   more as desired

FOR THE ICING

4 ounces cream cheese, softened

½ cup confectioners' sugar, plus more
   as needed

3 tablespoons Brown Sugar Simple
   Syrup (page 217)

1 teaspoon lemon zest

whole milk

NOTE

To save time in the morning, you can shred and drain the carrots ahead of time and then refrigerate them in an airtight container.

1. **MAKE THE PANCAKES:** Using the large holes of a box grater, shred the carrots. You should have about 1 cup. Place them in a clean towel and squeeze out as much moisture as possible and set the carrots aside.

2. In a medium bowl, whisk together the flour, granulated sugar, brown sugar, baking powder, baking soda, salt, cinnamon, ginger, and nutmeg.

3. In a large bowl, whisk together the milk, eggs, and vanilla until well combined. Add the carrots and mix to combine. Then add the dry ingredients and mix to combine. Cover the bowl and refrigerate about 30 minutes.

4. Meanwhile, **MAKE THE ICING:** In a small bowl, stir the cream cheese until it is uniformly soft and smooth. If needed, you can help the process along by microwaving the cream cheese for a few seconds at a time.

5. Add the confectioners' sugar, Brown Sugar Simple Syrup, and lemon zest and whisk until smooth. If you prefer a thinner icing, add milk, one teaspoon at a time. If the icing is too thin, add more confectioners' sugar, by the teaspoon.

6. To cook the pancakes, heat a large nonstick griddle or skillet over low heat. Add enough butter to coat the bottom. Working in batches, add ¼ cup batter for each pancake and sprinkle each with a few raisins. Cook until bubbles and little holes form in the pancake, 3 to 4 minutes. Turn and cook the other side. Add more butter to the pan as necessary.

7. Drizzle the icing over the warm pancakes and serve immediately.

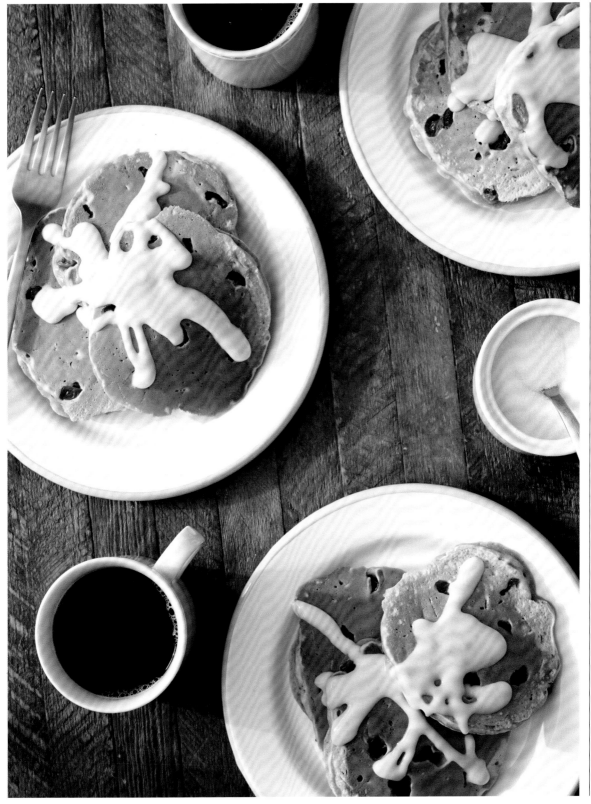

> The peace of God, which surpasses all understanding, will guard your hearts and your minds in Christ Jesus.
>
> PHILIPPIANS 4:7, ESV

In church I would often hear people pray, *Lord, please fill them with the peace that surpasses all understanding.* I knew what the phrase meant, and I believed it. I knew God was always there. Prayer had been a daily part of my life, in good times as well as times when I needed help. However, it wasn't until I experienced that peace in a moment of real crisis that I really did believe it with unyielding passion.

When I got pregnant in my late twenties, I was happy and scared all at once. The first eighteen weeks, I was so sick that I could barely get out of bed. I couldn't believe how incapacitated I was. Further into my second trimester, my symptoms began to subside. I traveled a little bit and continued working. When July approached, I had plans to unpack all my baby shower items, stock her room, clean out closets, and make freezer meals as my September due date drew nearer.

On July 5, after feeling a sort of contraction that never eased up, I was admitted to the hospital. For two days, doctors checked and rechecked me, wondering why the baby appeared to be fine in ultrasounds while the heart monitors showed steady movement instead of the levels of variation they hoped to see.

On the third morning, after another sleepless night, I was alone in the hospital room. I knew I was having small contractions, but I didn't want to tell anyone. I had spent two days and nights staring at the monitor, seeing no changes, yet I heard God say to me that I was going to deliver the baby.

I had always struggled to hear God's voice, partly because I was still working on trusting him completely. But at that moment, I knew. I may have cried a little bit, but I wasn't panicked. When the doctors told me that I needed a C-section, I felt sad that I could not carry her to term to give her all she needed. But from that point on, I was covered completely in God's peace. It certainly does surpass all understanding.

At no point did I think the baby was in danger. I knew the C-section was an emergency, although no one on the hospital staff used that word. I never thought about how surreal this all was. I just said, "Let's keep moving forward. What's next?" The doctors kept saying I could take my time and be upset. Instead, I kept saying, "You do not know my God."

Was Siena rushed away afterward? Yes. Did she have multiple blood transfusions and go through other difficult medical procedures? Yes. Did I struggle in the moments and weeks following? Yes. But I held on to what I experienced and learned in those moments in the hospital bed, that feeling of peace that made no worldly sense and God's still, small voice in the morning. Besides Siena, those moments have been the greatest gift of my life.

When we learn to hear that still small voice, it gives us the ability to access a deeper peace. It served me well when I battled thyroid cancer. This peace fell over me when I was wheeled into the operating room. There have been so many moments when I have anticipated pain or feared certain procedures or worried about the effects of recovery. Each time, God has met my anxiety with that same peace, and often the situation has proved to be less painful than imagined.

Each time I have chosen to surrender the situation that is beyond my control to God, he has delivered. That deliverance is there for you, should you choose to surrender.

Dear Lord, envelop me in your presence. Let your peace fall upon my heart, my home, and all that comes before me today. Help me to hear your still small voice in the wake of storms. Help me rest in your presence and take refuge in your arms. Let me know that you go before me, that you are already there.

Olive and Tomato Egg Bake

SERVES: 6 TO 8 | PREP: 15 MINUTES | COOK: 45 MINUTES | INACTIVE: 2 HOURS 40 MINUTES

As the holidays approach, menu planning is in full swing. It's a cross between a puzzle and a sports bracket. Which traditional dishes make the cut and when should they be served? One year, I noticed that with all the prep that goes into Christmas dinner, we were coming up short on the actual morning. Scrounging around for a bowl of cereal while we opened presents wasn't cutting it. This egg bake is easily prepared the night before, whether it's Christmas Eve or a random week in April. Just pop it in the oven after everyone has run down the stairs.

1 (12-ounce) package English muffins, halved and cut into 1-inch pieces (approximately 6 cups)

4 ounces shredded whole milk mozzarella cheese

1 cup halved cherry tomatoes

½ cup chopped Kalamata olives

8 large eggs

2 cups whole milk

½ cup whole milk Greek yogurt

1 teaspoon kosher salt

1 teaspoon ground black pepper

½ teaspoon onion powder

½ cup crumbled feta cheese

1½ teaspoons chopped fresh oregano

1. Coat a 9 by 13-inch baking dish with nonstick cooking spray.

2. Spread half of the English muffin pieces across the bottom of the dish. Sprinkle half each of the mozzarella, tomatoes, and olives over the muffin pieces. Add the remaining muffin pieces and top with the rest of the mozzarella, tomatoes, and olives.

3. In a medium bowl, whisk together the eggs, milk, yogurt, salt, pepper, and onion powder until well combined. Pour the egg mixture over the muffin mixture. Press gently on the muffin pieces so each is nicely coated with the egg mixture. Cover and refrigerate for at least 2 hours or overnight.

4. Preheat the oven to 375°F. Remove the pan from the refrigerator, uncover, and let come to room temperature.

5. Sprinkle with the feta and oregano. Bake until the top is lightly browned and the eggs are fully set when tested in the center with a toothpick, about 45 minutes. Let cool 10 minutes before serving.

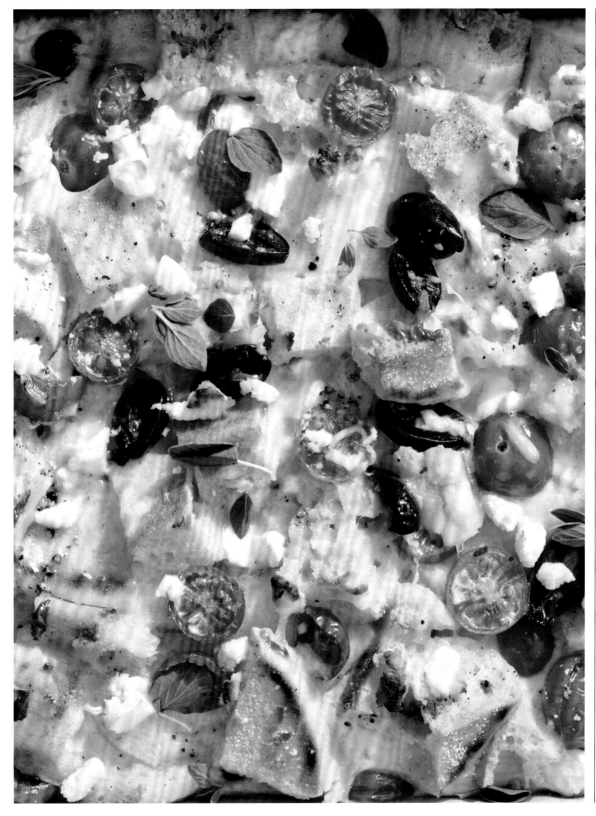

Have you ever been innocently watching television when the main character suffers through something tragic? Suddenly, instead of Netflix and chill, you're thinking of a situation you're trying to escape. Or maybe you dropped off your child at school and entered your workplace, and then suddenly became fearful of what the day will bring? Whether you meant to worry or not, it is there. You try to go about your day, but the fear has laid deep roots in your heart.

> God is our Refuge and Strength [mighty and impenetrable to temptation], a very present and well-proved help in trouble.
>
> PSALM 46:1, AMPC

Shortly after the first surgery to remove a cancerous cyst on my thyroid gland, my family and I went on our annual beach vacation. The timing was perfect. I knew another surgery and further treatments were on the horizon, but being at the beach was a wonderful reprieve.

One morning toward the end of our trip, I got up early to walk to the beach. I was praying about what lay ahead, asking God that the weight of my diagnosis wouldn't crush me when I returned home and that he would help me temper my feelings of worry and continue to live each day as he intended.

As I was praying, I saw the sunshine on the ocean. Behind me, though, were lots of ominous, dark gray clouds. At that moment, I felt God speak to me. He was asking me to keep my eyes on him and look forward, focusing on all the good that he put before me. We still had the rest of the summer to look forward to, and I had the blessing of this book to work on. If I looked behind me or focused on the impending storm, I surely would become anxious and distracted. *Why not surrender your fears to me?* he seemed to be asking. If I could daily be faithful in my surrender and move forward with my eyes on him, he would take care of the storm.

> Therefore we will not fear, though the earth should change and though the mountains be shaken into the midst of the seas,
> Though its waters roar and foam, though the mountains tremble at its swelling and tumult. Selah [pause, and calmly think of that]!
>
> PSALM 46:2–3, AMPC

As that day progressed, it never actually rained, and our beach day was perfect. Yet I could have looked at the dark clouds moving fast in the sky and thought the day was doomed. So many times, we proclaim the ending before something even begins. When we take our eyes off Jesus, we see the darkness of our circumstances and all that could go wrong. We see the relationship being ruined or the job we won't get or the looming illness or prognosis.

> There is a river whose streams shall make glad the city of God, the
>   holy place of the tabernacles of the Most High.
> God is in the midst of her, she shall not be moved; God will help her
>   right early.
>
> PSALM 46:4–5, AMPC

Instead of leaning in to our weakness, let us remind ourselves of his greatness. In the Bible, you see the word *Selah* after certain verses. The word basically means "pause and think of that." How often do we pause and let God's Word sink in? He is asking us to be still so he can fill our hearts with certainty instead of all the "what ifs." He can replace feelings of anxiety with his greatness and his promises.

Dear Lord, help me truly pause and think of all that you are. You are greater than my pain or disappointment. You are my great protector, my refuge, my high tower. You are the God who parted the Red Sea and raised the dead, the God of miracles. Help me know that you are in control. You see my worry and my concerns, and I lay them at your feet. Fill me with your peace, and steady my heart and mind.

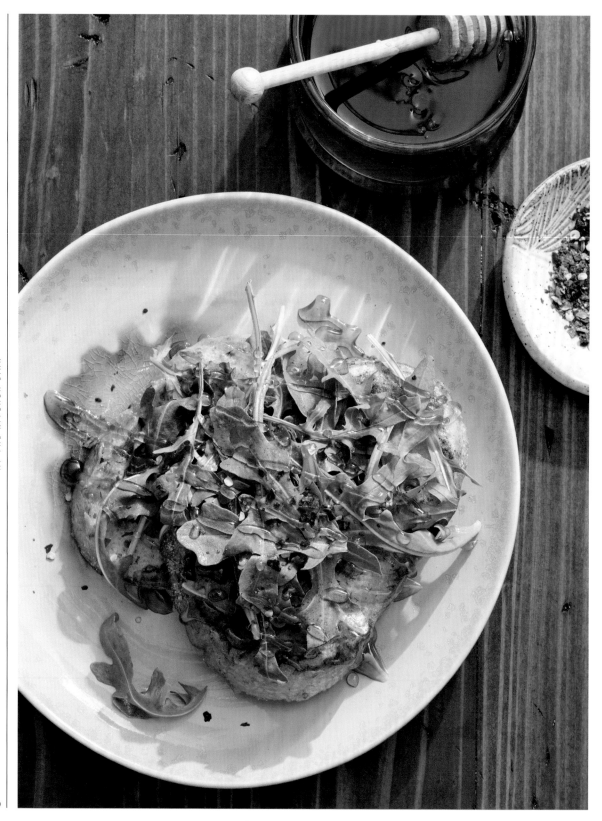

Savory French Toast

MAKES: 6 TOASTS | PREP: 5 MINUTES | COOK: 10 MINUTES

I have a confession: I am not big on breakfast. I usually pass up all the pastries, muffins, and sweet stuff. However, if I spy thick, crusty bread sitting on the counter, this savory version of French toast is my go-to. It's the best of both worlds: a fabulous piece of thick bread with egg, too, for protein. Instead of a sugary cinnamon vibe, you get the taste of an egg sandwich. For me, it almost beats out avocado toast. It's also a great way to serve breakfast for dinner.

3 large eggs

¼ cup heavy cream

½ teaspoon hot sauce

¼ teaspoon soy sauce

¼ teaspoon ground mustard

¼ teaspoon dried dill

¼ teaspoon kosher salt

⅛ teaspoon ground black pepper

⅛ teaspoon onion powder

1½ teaspoons unsalted butter

6 (¼-inch) slices from a round loaf of crusty Italian bread

Hot honey, for serving

Arugula, for serving (optional)

1. In a shallow bowl, whisk together the eggs, cream, hot sauce, soy sauce, mustard, dill, salt, pepper, and onion powder until well combined.

2. In a large skillet over medium heat, melt the butter, swirling the pan to coat the bottom.

3. Holding each slice of bread with a fork, dip the bread in the egg mixture, fully coating both sides and letting the excess egg mixture drip off. Cooking in batches, place the bread in the pan and cook, turning once, until golden brown on both sides, about 2 minutes per side.

4. Serve hot, drizzled with hot honey and topped with arugula (if using).

NOTE

I like to serve the pieces of bread with arugula when I have it on hand. I also like to sprinkle some red pepper flakes over the top for an added kick.

2
—
Mom Minute: Savoring Sanity

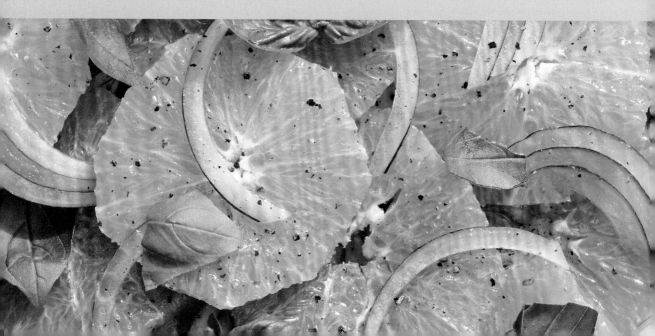

When we feel ourselves becoming overwhelmed, there is often a root cause beyond just being busy. We are taking care of everyone and balancing all the things, which adds to the pressure to keep up. It's no wonder we find ourselves gripping the edge of the kitchen sink, wondering how we'll make it to dinner-time. All too often, we find ourselves eating leftovers off of discarded breakfast plates or perhaps skipping lunch because we are trying to get one more thing done. Both of these habits lead us to being hungry, or perhaps "hangry" in both body and spirit.

Instead of stressing over the number of hours in the day or becoming resentful over the lack of "me" time, let me invite you to take a quick minute to step back from the edge and reheat your coffee. Those extra couple of minutes can revive and reset you. Perhaps making a Banana Coffee Whip (page 41), taking time to eat lunch, or having a Peanut Butter Fluff Date (page 45) midday can give you the boost you need to tackle the afternoon rush. Take some time to let God remind you that you've got this because your strength comes from him. You do not need to tackle this day alone.

They are to do good, to be rich in good works, to be generous and ready to share, thus storing up treasure for themselves as a good foundation for the future, so that they may take hold of that which is truly life.

1 TIMOTHY 6:18–19, ESV

When the seasons change, I clean out closets and rearrange items in our home. Summer into fall means bathing suits go to the attic to make room for sweaters. Soon, piles start to form with shirts and pants we've outgrown or items that we do not seem to have space for anymore. As I stared at those piles this year, I began thinking of the money we'd spent on all of it and how much turnover happens with material things. Sitting there, I contemplated the hard realization that everything I buy will, in fact, fade away.

We tend to think of our time here on earth as a chance to curate the life we envision. We want a certain type of home and lifestyle, and often

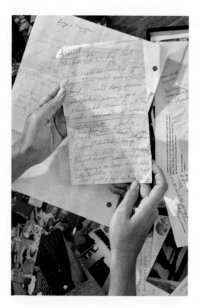

a certain status within our careers. We spend our efforts and resources, whether we have them or not, obtaining these things. Rarely, if ever, do we consider that when we pass away these things will be sold, donated, or even put in the trash. However, the work and effort you put into your family and your community will endure. The relationships we had with people and the interactions that left marks on their hearts will live beyond us. The time we spend raising our children, talking with them and guiding them, will shape who they become. These interactions will have ripple effects that cross generations and truly make a difference in ways the type of car in your driveway or the purse on your shoulder can't begin to touch.

The next time you find yourself restless and anxious, take inventory. What am I striving for? Society and social culture make it seem that without a certain aesthetic style in your home, you will not be happy. If you are not spending your time carpooling to every activity offered, your children will not be fulfilled. Without extra income from a side hustle, you are not contributing what you could to the family. Being able to scroll through the seemingly everyday lives of others can make us feel as though we aren't doing enough.

If you know, between you and the Lord, that you're putting your best foot forward, that is enough. Maybe you are not bringing up small children or parenting teenagers, but you're struggling through challenges in your marriage or as you attend school. Wherever you are in that season, know you are not falling short by being obedient. The co-worker to whom you minister, the child you comfort, the family you make meals for, the grandparents you visit—they all hold more weight than you imagine. Even though none of these actions do the slightest thing for the aesthetic of your life, these God-given tasks and interactions propel you forward. When you start to place higher value on these efforts, you will see your constant striving for more start to cease and your contentment rise.

———————

Dear Lord, please ease the overwhelming striving in my heart. Help me to see the importance in my everyday tasks and interactions. Help me to become hopeful in what each day may bring, instead of dreading what's to come. Fix and open my eyes to the blessings you place in front of me daily, helping my heart rejoice when recognizing them rather than mourn what I am without.

Off~the~Plate Raw Veggie Wrap

MAKES: 1 SANDWICH | PREP: 15 MINUTES

As a mom, I learned quickly that eating off your kid's plate is a fact, not a myth. When Siena started eating solid food, I found myself cutting up fruit and veggies for her every day. However, I noticed that because I was too busy moving from one task to the next, I would rarely eat during the day. I kept putting off eating until I finished this or that. Eventually, I discovered I could spend five minutes making something for myself and my whole day wouldn't fall apart. Plus, it would actually fuel me to be able to keep up with the demands of the day.

FOR THE CHICKPEA SPREAD

½ cup canned chickpeas, drained

2 tablespoon extra-virgin olive oil

2 tablespoons distilled white vinegar

½ teaspoon kosher salt

¼ teaspoon garlic powder

¼ teaspoon dried dill

Pinch of sugar

FOR THE WRAP

1 (10-inch) spinach tortilla

5 baby-cut carrots, chopped

¼ cup bean sprouts or
   2 lettuce leaves

4 thin slices avocado

6 thin slices cucumber

3 thin slices tomato, halved

⅛ teaspoon kosher salt

Pinch of ground black pepper

1 tablespoon Quick Pickled
   Red Onions (page 210)

2 thin slices dill Havarti cheese

1. **MAKE THE CHICKPEA SPREAD:** In a mini chopper or mini blender, pulse the chickpeas, oil, vinegar, salt, garlic powder, dill, and sugar until smooth.

2. **MAKE THE WRAP:** Place the tortilla on a flat work surface. Leaving a 1-inch border, spread the chickpea spread over the tortilla. Add the chopped carrots over the chickpea spread. In this order, layer the sprouts, avocado, cucumber, and tomato slices over the top. Sprinkle with salt and pepper, then finish with the pickled onions and cheese.

3. Fold in the sides of the wrap, then roll from the bottom as if you were making a burrito. Slice in half to serve.

NOTE

Make sure you have 10-inch tortillas on hand because the smaller ones tend to not work well. Or adapt this recipe to a sandwich with whatever bread you have on hand!

To save time, use 3 to 4 tablespoons of your favorite hummus instead of making the chickpea spread.

Swap out ingredients with something you already have. For example, any version of a 10-inch tortilla would work here, or try a different cheese.

To save this for later, wrap it in parchment paper and place in the fridge.

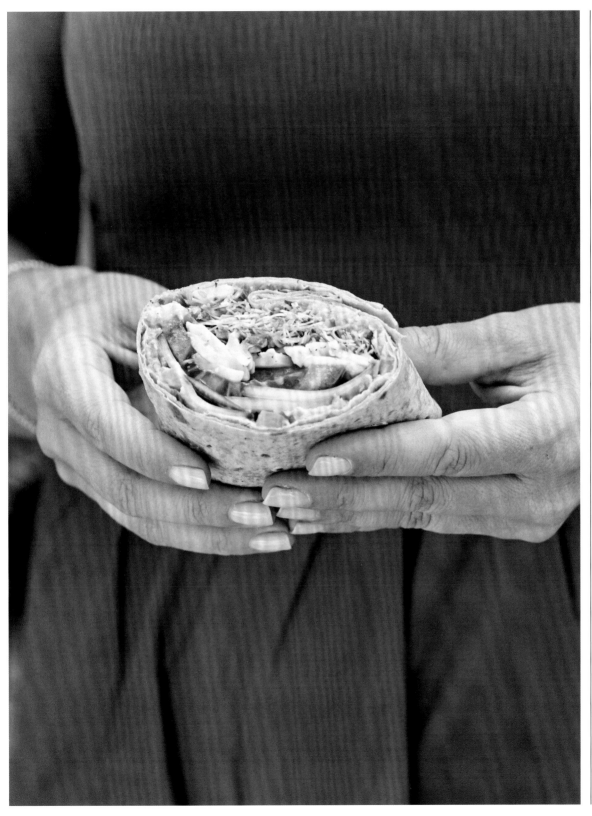

See, I am doing a new thing!
  Now it springs up; do you not perceive it?
I am making a way in the wilderness
  and streams in the wasteland.

ISAIAH 43:19

When I was walking through the lowest points of my postpartum depression, I struggled to keep up my relationships. I stopped having my family over for Sunday dinner, which was heartbreaking. I didn't go out with friends, because I felt as if I had nothing to say. I didn't want anyone to realize I couldn't relate to them. At my worst, I didn't care to hear from the people I loved. My heart was filled with frustration and anger. It wasn't self-care that I needed. It was God's care.

While the phrase "God's care" may not be considered trendy, it is what we truly need. It's popular to say that before you care for others, you should care for yourself and that you can't pour from an empty glass. But what happens when you don't have the energy or motivation to even look at the glass? Everything on social media told me I deserved long baths with a glass of wine, but those reminders just made me more frustrated. And I felt as though I was failing at one more thing if I fell asleep without doing a nine-step skin-care regimen.

On their own, none of these things are wrong or sinful. But God began to teach me that I was filling my glass with the wrong things. I pushed my career at the same rate I pushed Siena's stroller and tried to structure my days so they resembled Instagram posts. I was trying to find the time and finances for spa treatments and gym classes. But that wasn't what I needed this season. I was being fueled by comparison, and it had my glass overflowing with overwhelm.

When your relationship with yourself and with God is not right, you can't be of service to anyone else around you. How can you nourish a relationship when you're starving? You can't respond to God's calling, because

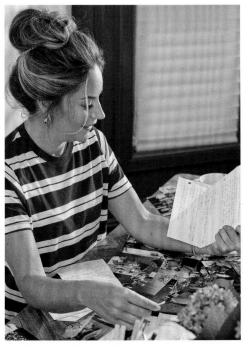

your heart is too broken to be listening. You can't hear his voice, because you are tuned in to the enemy's lies. Where do you need to begin the repairs? Maybe it's a relationship that needs healing, a marriage that needs tending, or a friendship that needs resolution. Or it might be a place in your heart that needs an apology or forgiveness. Are you trying to be everything to everyone, confronting and solving every issue and running so fast and pushing so hard that you don't even realize how far you have run away?

Let's get out of the wilderness and fill our glasses at the "streams in the wasteland."

Dear Lord, reveal to me what I need to let go of so I can be filled with the things you have for me. Give me the courage to surrender and start new. Help me not be resistant to your repairs. I pray that I feel the motivation to start somewhere and have faith that you will give me the strength to continue, trusting that you are my great provider, deliverer, and redeemer.

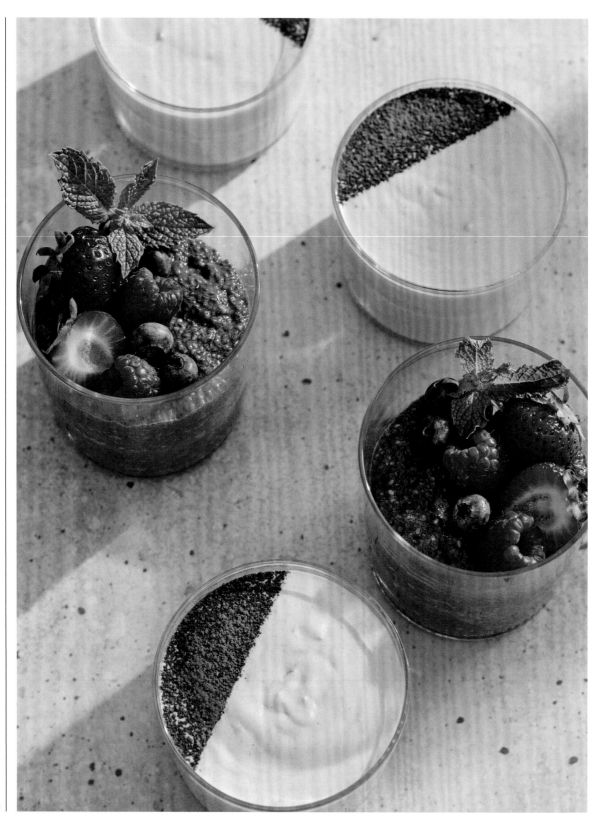

Coffee Chia Seed Pudding

SERVES: 1 | PREP: 5 MINUTES | INACTIVE: 4 HOURS

How many times can you reheat a cup of coffee before it's not worth drinking? After the first time, I'm over it. But dumping it down the drain is heartbreaking, and I'm also not into making coffee ice cubes. I love this coffee-spiked pudding, and it's a great way to use leftover coffee. It's also a healthy snack or easy breakfast.

¾ cup unsweetened almond milk

½ cup brewed coffee, cooled

2 tablespoons maple syrup

1 teaspoon natural cocoa powder

½ teaspoon ground cinnamon

½ cup chia seeds

Assorted berries, such as raspberries, blueberries, and strawberries, for serving (optional)

1. In a small bowl, combine the almond milk, coffee, maple syrup, cocoa powder, and cinnamon, stirring to dissolve the cocoa. Mix in the chia seeds.

2. Transfer to a small mason jar or other airtight glass container and refrigerate, stirring periodically, for at least 4 hours before serving. To serve, top with berries, if desired.

NOTE

If you have a larger jar with a tight lid, you can combine all the ingredients in the jar instead of using a bowl!

Banana Coffee Whip

SERVES: 2 | PREP: 10 MINUTES

Are bananas wasting away on your counter once again? I'm sure you bought the bunch with full intentions for each one—none of them being another loaf of banana bread. Before the bananas hit the garbage, try making yourself a batch of this Banana Coffee Whip. Save it in the fridge for up to a week and use it as the 3 P.M. pick-me-up that we all know we need!

1 ripe banana

½ cup heavy cream

2 tablespoons brewed coffee, cooled

1½ teaspoons maple syrup

1 teaspoon vanilla extract

⅛ teaspoon ground cinnamon

Cocoa powder, for serving (optional)

1. In a medium bowl, use a hand mixer on low speed to mash the banana. Add the cream, coffee, maple syrup, vanilla, and cinnamon. Increase to medium-high and beat until soft peaks form, about 4 minutes.

2. Spoon into two small ramekins or custard cups. Serve immediately or cover and chill overnight. Sprinkle with cocoa powder (if using) and serve chilled.

Breakfast Milk Smoothie

SERVES: 2 | PREP: 5 MINUTES

I have dumped one too many half-eaten bowls of cereal down the drain, but I knew there had to be a better way. Enter the Breakfast Milk Smoothie. The milk is already flavored, which means one less step for me. But for those who don't leave leftovers, here is a quick recipe that tastes just like it! Another thing I like to do is throw a scoop of my favorite protein powder into this mix as well!

2 cups unsweetened almond milk

1 ripe banana

½ cup Honey Nut Cheerios cereal

1 teaspoon maple syrup

1 cup ice

1. In a blender, combine the almond milk, banana, cereal, maple syrup, and ice and blend until smooth.

2. Pour into serving glasses and serve immediately.

NOTE

You can use your milk of choice in this recipe. It will slightly alter the flavor, but the thought behind this smoothie is that it should be reminiscent of what is leftover in your cereal bowl!

Another great cereal to use is corn flakes (any brand). If using corn flakes, add 1 teaspoon of honey instead of maple syrup.

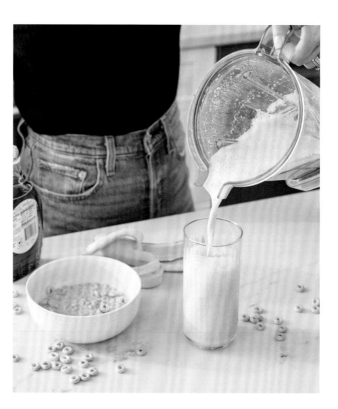

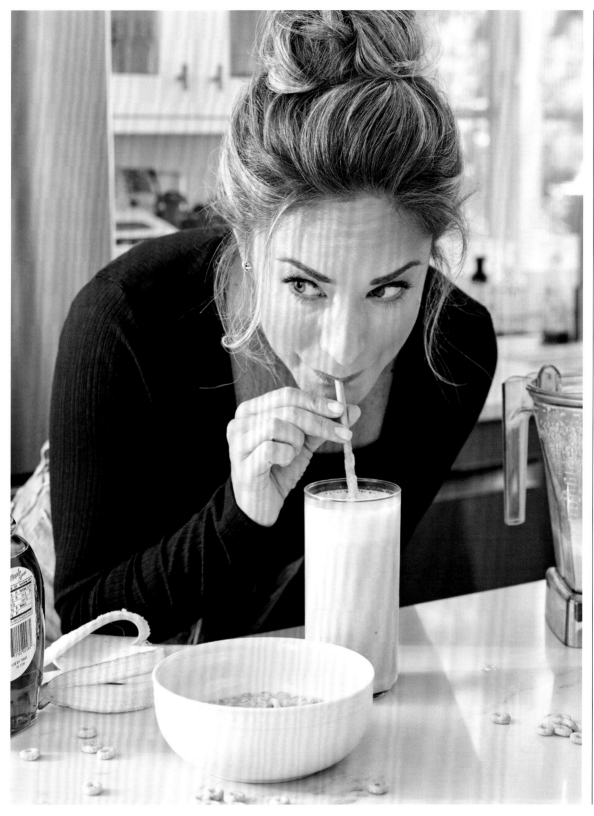

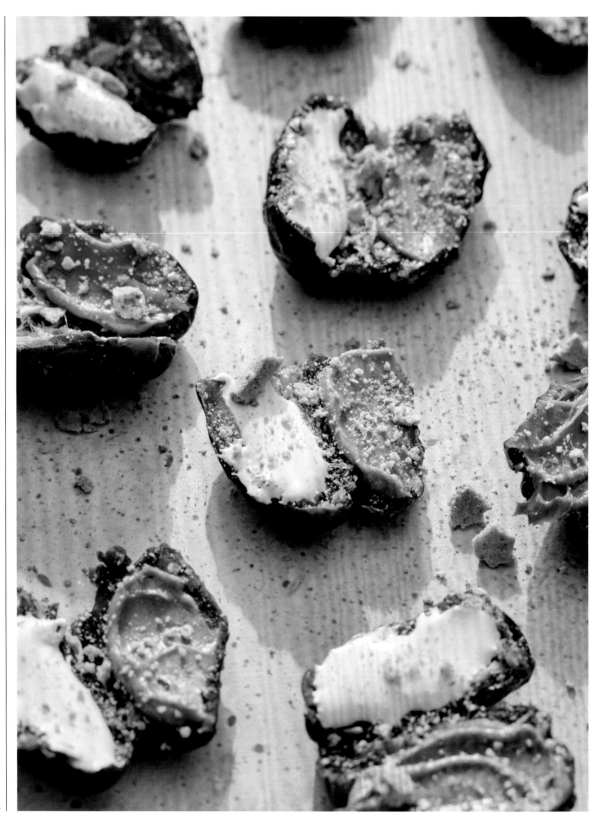

Peanut Butter Fluff Dates

Do you ever have days when you just need one minute to breathe before you go crazy? Inhale one of these dates and step back from the edge. I have these hiding in my fridge for just those occasions. Truth be told, they make great snacks for littles, if you feel like sharing.

24 large pitted dates

¼ cup creamy peanut butter

¼ cup marshmallow creme

1 rectangular graham cracker, crushed into crumbs

1. Line a small baking sheet with parchment paper.

2. Cut each date in half lengthwise, making sure to not cut all the way through, and gently open like a book. Fill one side of each date with about ½ teaspoon of peanut butter and the other side with an equal amount of marshmallow creme. Arrange on the baking sheet and sprinkle lightly with graham cracker crumbs.

3. Loosely cover the baking sheet with plastic wrap and refrigerate until set, about 30 minutes. Gently close each little date book to seal.

4. Line an airtight container with parchment paper. Carefully place the dates in the container and refrigerate for up to a week.

> The angel went to her and said, "Greetings, you who are highly favored! The Lord is with you."
>
> Mary was greatly troubled at his words and wondered what kind of greeting this might be. But the angel said to her, "Do not be afraid, Mary; you have found favor with God. You will conceive and give birth to a son, and you are to call him Jesus."
>
> LUKE 1:28–31

In my line of work, many people often wanted to know who I am. They'd ask, How did you get in the door? What are you famous for?

Before I did a television segment, they asked a series of questions for what they call a person's "lower thirds," the attributions that pop up on the screen underneath your name. The first few times I answered these questions, I felt self-conscious. I wasn't a published author of celebrity status or a classically trained chef. Did I really deserve to be where I was? At times, it seemed as though it didn't matter how hard I worked or how talented I may be—it simply wasn't ever going to be enough.

I imagine many of us feel that way at the end of the day. As we go through the stages of acceptance and rejection, we can lose sight of who we are. Soon we become judge and jury, believing that we are worth only what people are willing to give us. In a world obsessed with self-worth and identity, we can become so enmeshed with our jobs or families that we quickly lose sight of our God-given purpose.

> "I am the Lord's servant," Mary answered. "May your word to me be fulfilled." Then the angel left her.
>
> LUKE 1:38

What if Mary believed that she was truly just a peasant girl, unworthy of carrying the Son of God? As we go through life, we will no doubt hear many assessments and descriptions of ourselves. Some will be favorable and some perhaps unfair. We tend to focus and dwell on the negative more. Maybe we believe that we are too young or too old for what we want to achieve. Or maybe it seems like there is no place for us within our families, communities, or churches. We think we are not worth a certain job, so we don't apply. Those are lies crafted by Satan to keep us from moving forward as the person God has called us to be.

The angel was specific with Mary, stating that she was chosen, highly favored, and by no means alone—God was with her. He did not choose the queen or princess or someone with wealth or status. He chose Mary because he saw the purity of her heart. Her story reminds us that God uses the unlikely and that he doesn't measure us by the worldly standards that we measure ourselves.

Mary's simple response holds so much weight in my heart. She accepted, surrendered, and submitted herself to God's plan. Of course, it was not without trepidation or questions. When she went to visit her friend Elizabeth and tell her the news, Mary questioned why she was so favored that God would use her. Then the Holy Spirit spoke through Elizabeth:

Blessed is she who has believed that the
Lord would fulfill his promises to her!

LUKE 1:45

Who does Jesus say you are? My prayer is that I will surrender myself to his truth as Mary did and that I would lean in to who he says I am. That I would firmly believe he will fulfill his promises in my life, instead of believing in someone else's quantification of my worth. God knows my heart and has created me with purpose, as he has created you.

Dear Lord, I pray that I will tune in to your voice. That I would know how much you love me, despite what others may say. I am chosen.

Sicilian~Style Orange Salad

SERVES: 4 | PREP: 15 MINUTES

My grandmother always made orange salad on Christmas Eve. When I saw her making it for the first time, I remember commenting on how strange it was to put olive oil and so much pepper on oranges. She let me taste it and I realized why she loved it so much. Now, when Siena has leftover oranges, I almost always turn them into a smaller version of this salad for myself and smile. It may seem that it uses a lot of pepper, but anything less just tastes boring to me—and my grandma Rose was anything but boring!

4 large navel oranges, peeled, outer pith removed, and sliced into ¼-inch rounds

¼ small red onion, thinly sliced into half moons (about ¼ cup)

3 tablespoons extra-virgin olive oil

¼ teaspoon ground black pepper

⅛ teaspoon kosher salt

4 fresh basil leaves, torn

1. Arrange the orange slices on a serving platter and scatter the onions on top.

2. In a small bowl, whisk together the oil, pepper, and salt. Drizzle over the salad, add the torn basil, and serve at once.

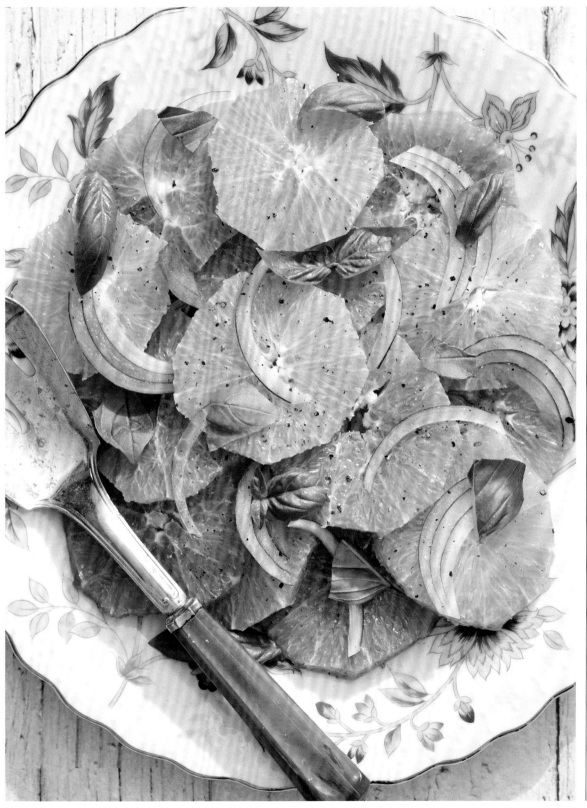

MOM MINUTE: SAVORING SANITY

3

Another Snack: Lunch and After~School Warriors

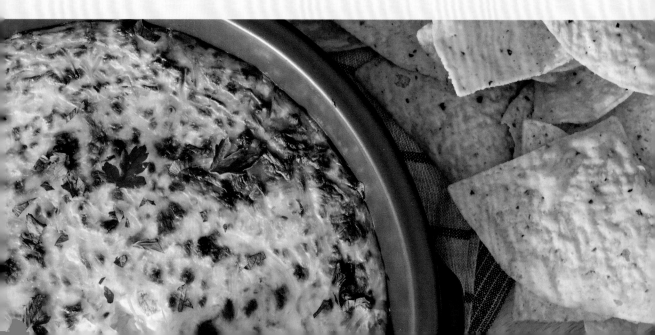

Everyone knows that making lunch can become a serious chore. Day in and day out, we rack our brains trying to pack something new and exciting, only to have our little ones bring it home untouched. It is the quintessential mundane task, something that seems tedious or of little importance. However, the small ways in which we serve our families, communities, and workplaces are acts of obedience. They help lay the foundation that a home and community is built upon. These tasks are acts of love and care, which serve to help cultivate long-term and meaningful relationships.

Sharing Pumpkin Chocolate Chip Cookies (page 64) after school could lead to a conversation with your kids about their day. Having a whole platter of Italian Sub–Inspired Stuffed Bread (page 74) on a Friday night for your teens and their friends to devour is a way for you to provide a friendly space. Let this chapter show you that the mundane is in fact marvelous. That star-shaped peanut butter and jelly sandwich is kingdom work!

A Note on Kids' Plates

So often, I am asked about how I get Siena to eat certain foods. The truth is she is just as particular as any other kid out there. Yes, she eats crispy broccoli and string beans, and she loves the flounder recipe. She even often requests sushi because of her love of seaweed. However, she refuses to eat peanut butter and jelly, grilled cheese, and cheese in general—unless my dad is hand pulling mozzarella. Go figure.

Our dinner table can be tense and exasperating at times. But there are some tactics I used early on that seemed to help her at least give foods a try. I hope sharing them helps spur ideas of your own. Most important, realize you are not doing anything wrong if your child doesn't eat all their vegetables. They go through stages, phases, mood swings, and everything in between. While your efforts may prove fruitless (pun intended), they are not in vain. Your child's eating habits do not correlate with whether or not you are a good parent.

Emergency Mac and Cheese

On nights where I know the sell is going to be a hard one, I cut my losses up front. I make a box of mac and cheese, keeping it on the stove, in the event that she cannot stomach the main part of the meal. You may think that's giving in or creating an out. Will she manipulate the system and just always reject the food for the mac and cheese? Sure, it is possible. However, I think you can tell the difference between a real food aversion and, well, not. I do not believe in forcing her to eat something she is truly gagging on. Kids have likes and dislikes just like adults, and that is okay.

Another way I use the mac and cheese is by putting a little bit on her plate so there is a sure bet. When she gets to the table, she sees something on her plate that she loves. Then she is less apt to be overwhelmed by the things on her plate that she's not so excited about.

Deconstruction

Sometimes kids need to be introduced to foods in a different presentation than an adult. For example, sausage and peppers. At first glance, they may not be palatable all together. However, your child may like sliced raw peppers and the sausage cut up with dipping sauce on the side. Whatever the dinner I'm making for our family, I have always tried to deconstruct it for Siena. If I am not sure she will like the pasta sauce, I give her plain pasta. Then I let her spoon on the sauce or dip the pasta in the sauce herself. When we had tacos, I served her all the ingredients separately. Then I graduated to plain quesadillas, and so on.

Eat with Them

Even besides dinner, I would try to make sure to sit and eat with Siena. As she was exploring solid food, I saw what was on my plate was her biggest influence. That is how Siena started eating salad. We were eating lunch in the playroom while watching *Mickey Mouse Clubhouse*, and she grabbed a piece of lettuce off my plate. I froze. I had not thought of giving her lettuce for a myriad of reasons. Now she loves salad, specifically with my balsamic vinaigrette dressing and chopped apples. Even now, when she's hit a stage where she is less willing to do the "try me" bite, she is still inquisitive. She will ask what I am eating or what it tastes like. Hopefully one day she will ask to try some herself.

It can be hard to sit and eat dinner. You are getting up a hundred times during the meal. At breakfast time, you are most likely packing lunch bags at the same time. But even sharing snacks with your children in the car or at the park is valuable. They'll see you munching on carrots or apples, and most of the time they will be inclined to at least try them. Sometimes we forget that they truly are watching us, although perfection in any area is not what we should strive for. It is great to do little things here and there purposely for their benefit.

Include Them

Where it is appropriate, have your children help with food prep. If they aren't helping specifically with dinner, let them play with the ingredients. Let them help you measure and dump when making banana bread. It is also great for fine motor skills, along with hand-eye coordination. I found Siena was also more likely to try something when we had made it together.

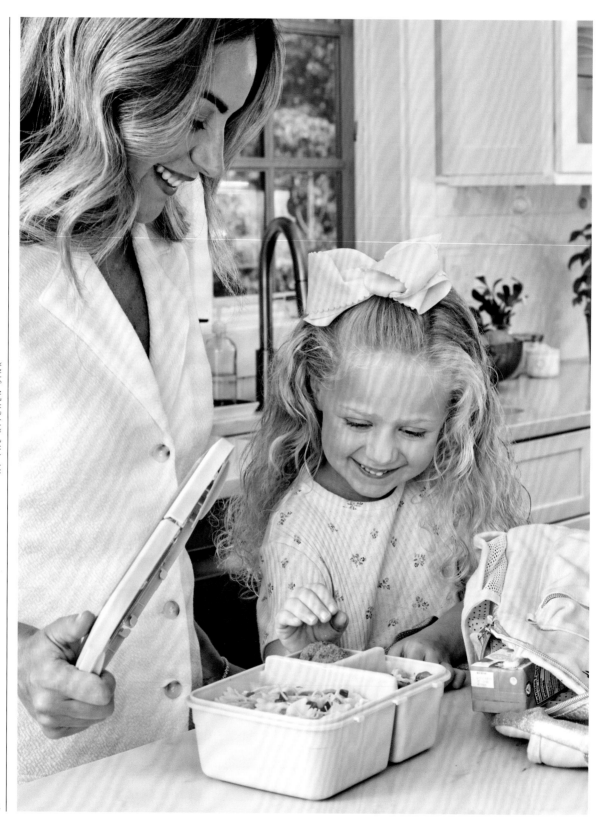

Now that Siena is a bit older, she loves to set herself up at the kitchen island with a mixing bowl. She will take my scraps and mix them up. Of course, this doesn't mean I am letting her play with knives or cayenne pepper. I make sure the ingredients and tools are safe.

I also like to bring her along to the grocery store and let her choose. There have been plenty of times she has opted to try a new fruit or healthy snack. Or she picks out a dinner entrée for one night during the week and she is quite proud of herself. Sometimes we forget how rarely kids get to make their own choices. As they age, they want a bit more independence and a voice. This is one great way to give them that chance.

"Let Me Reintroduce Myself"

One rule I have stuck to is never making anything extinct from the table. Just because Siena doesn't like it one day doesn't mean she won't go for it the next time she sees it. Unfortunately, this works the other way too. I can't tell you how many times she has been in love with apples only to shun them for the next two weeks. Other times, she has surprised me by going for a meatball when she swore she would never touch one again.

Please note that I am not a trained dietitian or anything of that nature. I do not specialize in nutrition or feeding. I am just a mom who found what worked for my child. If you suspect your child is having physical or emotional issues related to eating and food, please consult your doctor. Also, please use your discretion in implementing any of these strategies. Keep in mind your child's age, temperament, and personal needs, which you are attuned to.

> The LORD will guide you continually,
> giving you water when you are dry
> and restoring your strength.
> You will be like a well-watered garden,
> like an ever-flowing spring.
>
> ISAIAH 58:11, NLT

In a moms groups or among friends, we often look at one another and ask, How do you do it all? Recently, I got the feeling that I needed to ask a more fundamental question: What *is* my "all"? And who truly asked me to do the things I've put on my daily list?

Brian and I would often get into arguments after I'd listed all that I was doing. Sometimes he would stare at me blankly and say, "Well, no one is making you do that." That response set me on fire—and still does—but Brian had a point. I didn't need to continue doing anything that was putting me over the edge. Maybe we didn't need the laundry done, even if it was laundry day. Or we could have ordered takeout instead of me insisting on starting homemade lasagna at 6:30 P.M. And if a task absolutely *did* have to get done, I could ask him to help me with it.

When we talk about trying to do it all, we often think the solution is finding some kind of perfect balance. I think it's more about having the ability to know when it's time to take inventory of our family routines and capacities and then bringing them to the Lord while accepting that life looks different for everyone. Instead of becoming anxious in the slower or uncertain seasons, I surrender to him and trust that he is able to open doors without me hustling my way through.

> For the vision is yet for the appointed time;
> It hurries toward the goal and it will not fail.
> Though it delays, wait for it;
> For it will certainly come, it will not delay long.
>
> HABAKKUK 2:3, NASB

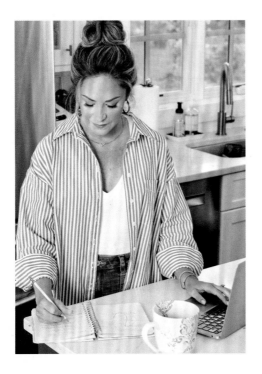

Some days my life looks like facilitating the production of a photo shoot, fielding phone calls, and writing emails. Other days it's all about school drop-off, the grocery store, Barbie dolls, and loads of laundry in between.

There are times when God asks us to run and others when he asks us to walk. Then there are times when he asks us to just sit and wait with him. We have to be willing to participate however he asks, with open arms and minds. I struggled to slow down, always wanting to check all the boxes. Now I bring it to him a lot sooner. I ask him to calm my anxious, ambitious heart when need be, and to fan the flames of motivation when a dream truly does come from him.

Dear Lord, help me be content in the season that lies ahead, knowing you have not forgotten about me. You know the desires of my heart. I am not without purpose or plan. Help me seek your direction in all things, being content in the in-between and expectant and obedient as I wait. I pray that I would find joy in the journey rather than satisfaction in the physical race.

Chocolate Cherry Bars

MAKES: 9 BARS | PREP: 15 MINUTES | COOK: 35 MINUTES | INACTIVE: 15 MINUTES

Chocolate-covered cherries, one of my favorite candy treats, inspired these indulgent-tasting, oat-rich bars. Having a batch in the fridge ensures that a great midday snack always is within easy reach. They also work great in lunch boxes!

2½ cups quick-cooking rolled oats

1½ cups puffed rice cereal

½ cup coconut sugar

1½ teaspoons baking powder

¼ teaspoon ground cinnamon

⅛ teaspoon kosher salt

1 ripe banana

2 large eggs

½ cup unsweetened almond milk

1½ teaspoons maple syrup

1 teaspoon almond extract

½ cup dried cherries, roughly chopped

¾ cup milk chocolate chips

MORE TO SHARE RECIPE

1. Preheat the oven to 350°F. Line the bottom and sides of an 8- or 9-inch square pan with parchment paper, leaving a 1-inch overhang on two sides.

2. In a medium bowl, stir together the oats, rice cereal, coconut sugar, baking powder, cinnamon, and salt until well combined.

3. In a large bowl, mash the banana, then add the eggs, milk, maple syrup, and almond extract and stir until well combined. Add the oat mixture. Using a rubber spatula, mix until well combined, then fold in the cherries and chocolate chips.

4. Transfer the mixture to the prepared pan. Use the spatula to firmly press it into an even layer. Bake until set, about 35 minutes.

5. Using the parchment paper handles, carefully lift the bars out of the pan and transfer to a wire rack. Let cool for 15 minutes. Transfer to a cutting board and, using a sharp knife, cut into nine squares. Let cool completely. The bars can be refrigerated in an airtight container for up to 5 days.

NOTE

Boost the nutritional benefits by adding a few tablespoons of ground flaxseed to the mix. Cacao chips also work well.

If you do not like dried cherries, try substituting them with dried cranberries.

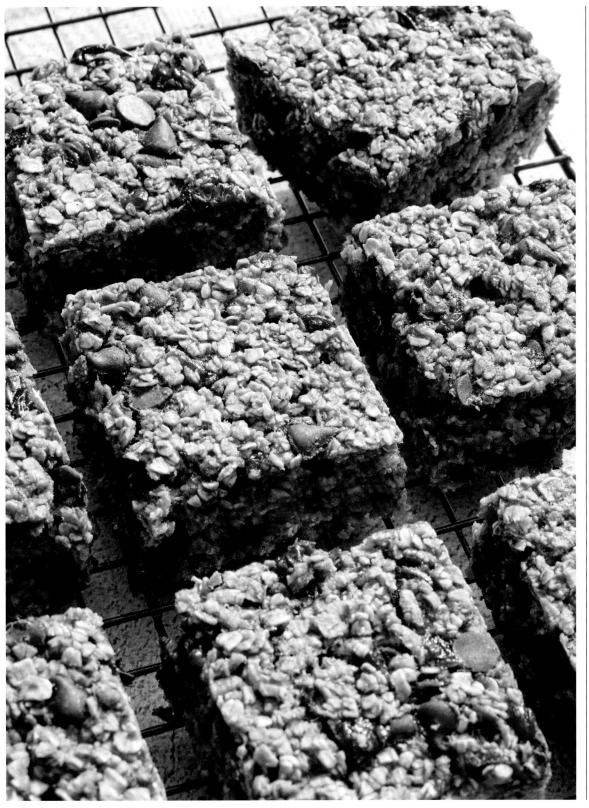

Fruit Snacks Trail Mix

Packing school lunches is no easy task. Over time, the job gets tedious and monotonous. What is even more challenging is getting a good amount of protein in kiddos throughout the day. I consider myself lucky that Siena actually likes cashews, which makes trail mix an option. (If she would eat a PB&J or grilled cheese, that would be wonderful. But I digress . . .) The addition of fruit snacks makes this a fun option for kids, while a backdrop of warm spices makes it fun for adults too.

3 tablespoons unsalted butter, melted

1 teaspoon honey

¼ teaspoon ground cinnamon

¼ teaspoon ground cardamom

1½ cups raw whole cashews

1 cup coarsely chopped pecans

1 cup fruit snacks (anything will work here)

½ cup chocolate-covered cranberry or raisin bites

1 cup unsweetened coconut chips

1. Preheat the oven to 350°F. Line a sheet pan with parchment paper.

2. In a large bowl, stir together the butter, honey, cinnamon, and cardamom. Add the cashews and pecans and stir to coat them with the mixture.

3. Spread the nuts evenly on the sheet and bake until mostly dried out and golden, about 12 minutes. Cool completely.

4. Transfer the nuts to a large bowl and add the fruit snacks, cranberry bites, and coconut chips. Toss gently to combine. Store in an airtight container at room temperature for up to 1 week.

Do not be afraid, for I am with you;
    I will bring your children from the east
    and gather you from the west.
I will say to the north, "Give them up!"
    and to the south, "Do not hold them back."
Bring my sons from afar
    and my daughters from the ends of the earth—
everyone who is called by my name,
    whom I created for my glory,
    whom I formed and made.

ISAIAH 43:5–7

Have you ever found yourself thinking that you wish you were living, or raising children, during a different time?

Every other day, it seems we are confronted with news stories where the unimaginable has become reality. Even if we're not the type who stay glued to the television, our phones and social feeds will fill us in. While some of these situations are a world away, we can't help becoming emotionally involved. As we try to keep our homes in order and worry about those we love, the lack of control over outside situations can begin to feel, well, scary. Everyday tasks such as going grocery shopping or dropping off your children at school start to feel like a life-or-death decision. It can be paralyzing and stifling.

I think often about the story of Esther. She became the queen at a time when her new husband, the king, had issued a decree for all the Jews to be killed. Esther had favor with the king, but her people were suffering. When her uncle, Mordecai, pleaded with her to approach the king, she was afraid. Mordecai said to her,

And who knows but that you have come to your royal position for such a time as this?

ESTHER 4:14

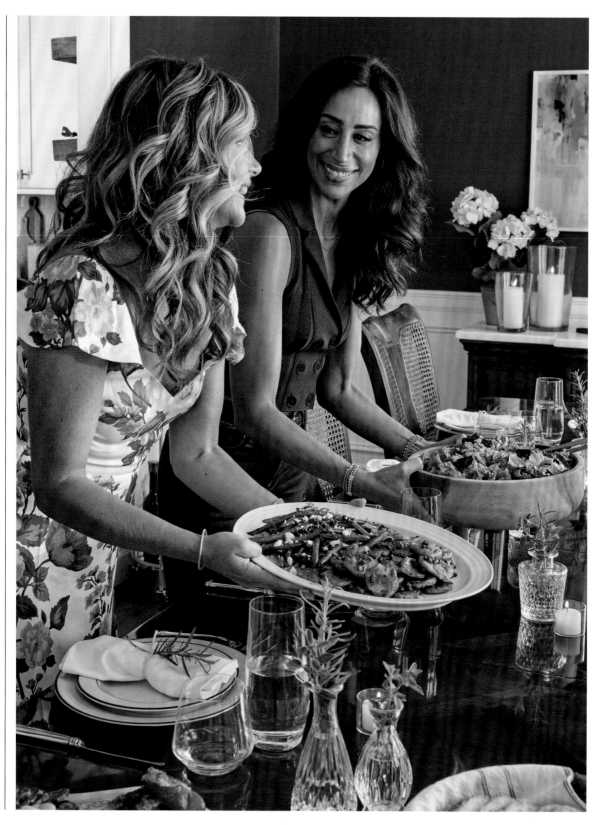

I often joke that I was meant to live during the 1960s because I love the dresses, listening to Dean Martin, and watching *That Girl* with my mom. But I have to consider that I am meant to be Siena's mom—for such a time as this. I am meant to be a part of our school and community—for such a time as this. Even when I walk through the doors of the cancer center, who knows . . . someone may need the prayer I'm praying then. Each time I drop Siena off at school, I cover the parking lot in prayer. Just like Esther, I will cover with prayer the kingdom I am in and walk with the power of the Lord within me.

We need to remind ourselves of the powerful God we serve. He is the same yesterday, today, and forever. Our circumstances change, but he does not. He is the same God who delivered the Israelites from Egypt. He is the same God who shut the mouths of the lions in the den and who walked in the fiery furnace with Shadrach, Meshach, and Abednego. Through God's goodness, that power lives within us. When we remind ourselves of this, we can face our days less afraid of what is to come.

———————————

Dear Lord, thank you for creating me for such a time as this. For equipping me in ways that only you can. Thank you for your endless protection and provision. I pray that you will continue to go before me and my loved ones. Cover my community, my workplace, my church, and anywhere else my feet may bring me. Thank you for calling me by name!

Pumpkin Chocolate Chip Cookies

MAKES: 2 DOZEN COOKIES | PREP: 15 MINUTES | COOK: 12 MINUTES | INACTIVE: 20 MINUTES

When it comes to baking, I can lay claim to more disasters than triumphs, thanks to all the precise measurements that can seem fussy at times. But these cookies are one of my greatest creations. Almost cakelike—the perfect consistency for me. The pumpkin taste is deliciously subtle, not at all reminiscent of the pumpkin spice that plagues us in the fall. (Yes, I said it!) Getting Siena to eat something with pumpkin in it also feels like a win. Makes it healthy, right?

2½ cups all-purpose flour

1 teaspoon baking soda

1 teaspoon salt

1 cup (2 sticks) unsalted butter, softened

¾ cup granulated sugar

¾ cup packed light brown sugar

2 large eggs

½ cup and 1 tablespoon pumpkin puree

1 tablespoon maple syrup

1 teaspoon vanilla extract

½ teaspoon cinnamon

2 cups milk chocolate chips

MORE TO SHARE RECIPE

NOTE

Alternatively, you can scoop out cookie dough mounds and transfer them to a ziplock bag and store in the freezer for up to 2 months. When you later want to bake them, first place frozen mounds on a parchment-lined baking sheet and thaw in the refrigerator for at least 2 hours. Bake at 375°F until golden brown around the edges but still soft in the center, 12 to 14 minutes.

1. Preheat the oven to 375°F. Line three baking sheets with parchment paper.

2. In a medium bowl, whisk together the flour, baking soda, and salt until well combined. Set aside.

3. In a large bowl, use a hand mixer on low speed to beat the butter and both sugars until smooth and creamy, about 3 minutes. Add the eggs, one at a time, beating well after each addition. Add the pumpkin, maple syrup, vanilla, and cinnamon; mix to combine. Stop the mixer, add the dry ingredients, and mix until just combined. Add the chocolate chips and fold to combine.

4. Cover the bowl and refrigerate, about 20 minutes.

5. Using a 3-tablespoon cookie scoop, scoop the dough onto the pans, spacing each cookie 2 inches apart.

6. Bake until the cookies are golden brown at the edges, about 12 minutes. Let them sit on the pan for 5 minutes, then carefully transfer them to a cooling rack to cool completely. Store in an airtight container for up to 5 days.

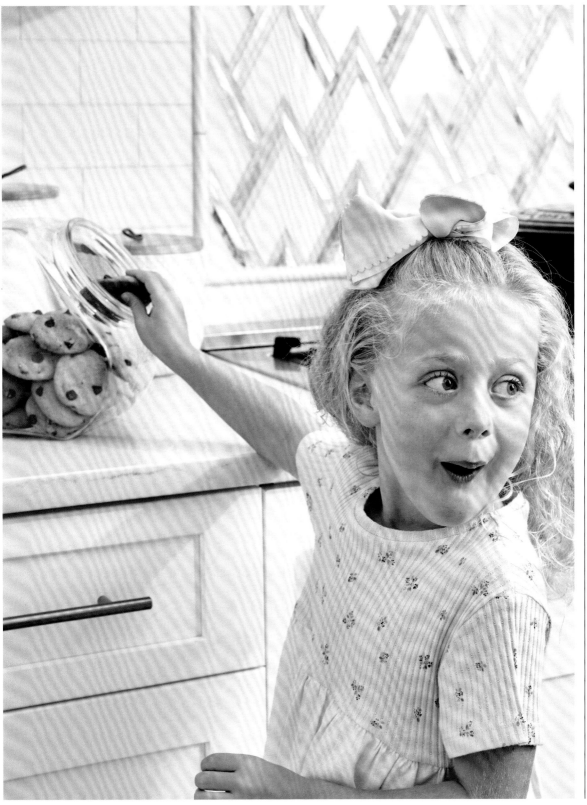

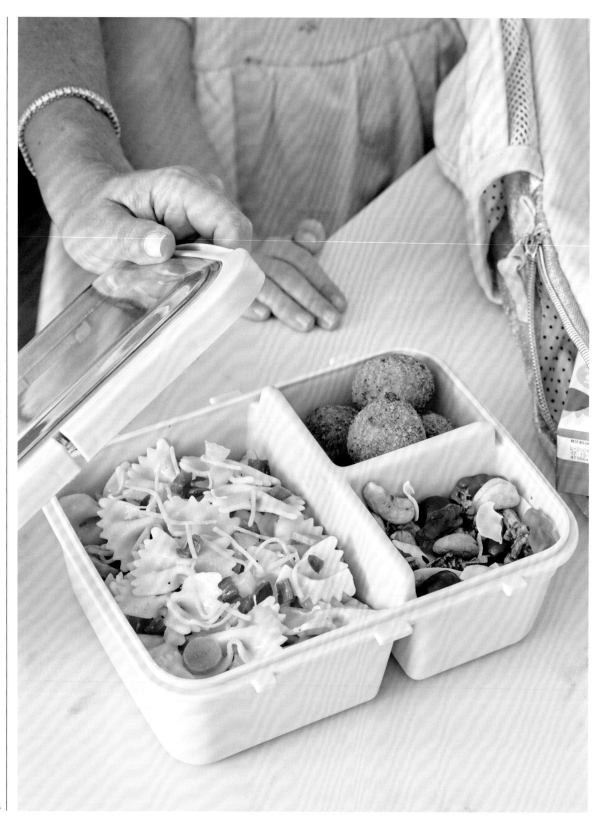

Honey Mustard Pasta Salad

SERVES: 4 TO 5 | PREP: 15 MINUTES | COOK: 15 MINUTES | INACTIVE: 15 MINUTES

Pasta salad recipes are wonderfully versatile, and the ingredients are easily changed by season, whim, and what's on hand. Once you have a great dressing, you can play around with the ingredients. I love traditional pasta salads tossed in pesto or a light, well-seasoned vinaigrette. This version is colorful with a tangy, sweet honey mustard vinaigrette. I use bow tie pasta, which makes it even more appealing to Siena.

1 tablespoon plus 1 teaspoon kosher salt

1 pound farfalle pasta

½ cup extra-virgin olive oil

3 tablespoons apple cider vinegar

2 tablespoons honey

1½ teaspoons Dijon mustard

1 garlic clove, minced

¼ teaspoon ground black pepper

1 large red bell pepper, seeded and cut into ¼-inch pieces (about 1 cup)

1 large yellow bell pepper, seeded and cut into ¼-inch pieces (about 1 cup)

2 small carrots, cut into thin rounds (about ½ cup)

1½ teaspoons finely diced shallot

¾ cup shredded mild Cheddar cheese, for serving

1. Bring a large pot of water to a boil. Add 1 tablespoon of the salt and the pasta. Cook until al dente, 11 to 12 minutes; drain and transfer to a large bowl.

2. Meanwhile, in a small bowl, make the vinaigrette by whisking together the oil, vinegar, honey, mustard, garlic, the remaining 1 teaspoon of salt, the pepper, and 1 tablespoon of cold water until well combined.

3. While the pasta is still warm, add the red and yellow peppers, carrots, and shallots to the pasta and gently toss to combine.

4. Pour the vinaigrette over the pasta and toss until everything is well coated. Let stand for 15 minutes, stirring every 5 minutes. When it's time to serve, gently fold in the cheese.

NOTE

Dress the pasta salad while it is still warm. If it won't be served right away, add about ⅔ of the dressing, reserving the rest to add just before serving.

If you have leftovers, give the pasta salad a little refresh by adding a splash more olive oil, salt, and pepper and toss again before serving.

> *When they measure themselves by themselves and*
> *compare themselves with themselves, they are not wise.*
>
> 2 CORINTHIANS 10:12

Do you find that you're quick to give other people the benefit of the doubt, but struggle to give yourself the same grace? I get it. When you feel tired or overwhelmed or when you've just snapped at a co-worker or screamed at your kids and are left to stare at the wreckage, the last thing you give yourself is grace. It feels more natural to give yourself a life sentence without parole.

Many times we feel the weight of failure because we measure ourselves based on comparisons. You feel like you failed because your house isn't as clean as your friend's across the street. Most nights, she also makes dinner from scratch, so surely she must be a better wife or mom. The women you follow on social media work out daily and manage to not overeat. Surely they have more friends, they deserve to lead a healthier life. So often I hear people, myself included, express frustration or sadness over not being able to do more.

It is good to have goals and aspirations, but when they become the measure of our success, they quickly turn into idols. We can get stuck in a cycle of striving and falling short, rather than thriving and moving forward.

> *Those who live according to the flesh have their minds set on*
> *what the flesh desires; but those who live in accordance with*
> *the Spirit have their minds set on what the Spirit desires. The*
> *mind governed by the flesh is death, but the mind governed*
> *by the Spirit is life and peace.*
>
> ROMANS 8:5–6

Our God-given path will never look like someone else's, but that doesn't mean we won't be successful. Would you tell your hardworking parents that they weren't successful because they didn't land on the cover of *Forbes*? Would you tell your friend who spends her time volunteering that her weekend wasn't Instagram worthy? Probably not! Why, then, are we so quick to judge ourselves by such harsh standards?

There are days when I still struggle with feelings of failure. I worry that I'm not reading enough with Siena or that I didn't spend enough time with her. I fall short and lose my temper with multiple people over the course of any given day. I come close to missing a deadline, forget to text someone back, and run out of time and energy to exercise. Led by stress, I eat the second piece of cake. The list goes on and on.

We do not need to stay stuck in a perceived mistake, whatever it may be. We can it give to God and say, *What can you make of this?* Let him be the redeemer, the deliverer.

> Therefore, there is now no condemnation for those who are in Christ Jesus, because through Christ Jesus the law of the Spirit who gives life has set you free from the law of sin and death.
>
> ROMANS 8:1–2

Dear Lord, please stand in the gaps where I feel like I am not enough. I bring my sin, frustration, and shortcomings to you, laying them at your feet. Thank you for giving your life so I can live free from shame and sin. Please cover me in your grace as I walk through my days. Help me not to feel condemned or forsaken. I know that you are with me regardless of shortcomings. Thank you that your mercies are new each and every day.

Crispy Broccoli and Cheese Rice Balls

MAKES: ABOUT 50 BITES | PREP: 35 MINUTES | COOK: 15 MINUTES

Crispy on the outside and cheesy on the inside—what's not to love? These little bites are a great way to help get kids to happily eat more vegetables. They take a little time, but they're worth it. You can grab them and go during busy weekdays.

1 cup long grain white rice

1 tablespoon extra-virgin olive oil

1 tablespoon minced garlic

1 cup riced broccoli

¼ teaspoon kosher salt, plus more for finishing

¼ teaspoon garlic powder

¼ teaspoon paprika

⅛ teaspoon ground black pepper

½ cup finely shredded Cheddar cheese

½ cup freshly grated Parmigiano-Reggiano cheese

4 large eggs

1¼ cups Italian-style bread crumbs, divided

½ cup all-purpose flour

Avocado oil or canola oil for frying

NOTE

During dredging, the egg may get a bit thick. If so, add 1 teaspoon cold water and beat the egg again to loosen it.

The second batch may cook more quickly. Adjust the heat so they don't get too brown before they're cooked in the center.

The recipe can be made up to 2 hours ahead of time, up to the dredging process, then covered and refrigerated. Let the rice balls stand at room temperature for 10 minutes before frying.

If you can't find riced broccoli, you can make your own by pulsing broccoli florets in the food processor until they reach a ricelike consistency.

1. Cook the rice according to package instructions. Set aside to cool.

2. In a large sauté pan over medium heat, warm the olive oil. Add the garlic and cook until fragrant, 1 minute. Add the riced broccoli and salt and stir to coat in the oil. Add the garlic powder, paprika, and pepper and stir. Continue to cook, stirring, until the broccoli is tender, 2 to 3 minutes. Set aside to cool for 5 minutes.

3. Add the broccoli mixture, rice, and both cheeses to a large bowl and toss to combine. Add two eggs and ¼ cup of bread crumbs and mix well to combine; the mixture should start to bind and become uniform.

4. Using three large shallow bowls, set up a dredging station: put remaining 1 cup of bread crumbs in one bowl and flour in another. Crack the remaining 2 eggs into the third bowl and whisk lightly to mix.

5. Using a small cookie scoop (approximately 2 teaspoons), portion the rice mixture and, with the palms of your hands, lightly roll them into small balls.

6. Coat each ball with flour, shaking off any excess. Next, coat with the egg and then the bread crumbs. Arrange on a large baking sheet.

7. Use a paper towel to lightly wipe any residue from the sauté pan used to cook the broccoli mixture. Add avocado oil to a depth of ½ inch and heat until a few bread crumbs dropped in the oil sizzle immediately.

8. Cooking in batches, gently add the coated rice balls to the hot oil. Cook, turning as needed, until golden brown all over, 1 to 2 minutes per side. After they're cooked, transfer to a paper towel–lined plate and sprinkle with salt. Serve immediately.

Ultimate English Muffin Pizzas

MAKES: 6 MINI PIZZAS | PREP: 6 MINUTES | COOK: 10 MINUTES

Some of my core memories of growing up are when my mom would make me pizza muffins, pour me a glass of fruit punch, and let me sit in the family room at my little blue table. I would watch all the Christmas cartoons while eating this dish. The crunch of the English muffin and the gooey cheese melted into my mom's tomato sauce was the ultimate comfort food. I still have the VHS tape of those cartoons, by the way. It is one of my most prized possessions. And yes, I still eat pizza muffins while watching those cartoons alongside my daughter now.

4 tablespoons unsalted butter, melted

1 teaspoon chopped garlic

½ teaspoon dried parsley

¼ teaspoon kosher salt

Pinch of ground black pepper

3 English muffins, split in half

½ cup Easy Marinara Sauce (page 111)

½ cup shredded low-moisture whole milk mozzarella cheese

1. Preheat the oven to 375°F. Line a rimmed baking sheet with parchment paper.

2. In a small bowl, stir together the butter, garlic, parsley, salt, and pepper.

3. Place the English muffins, cut-side up, on the prepared baking sheet. Brush the cut sides with the butter mixture, then add 1 tablespoon of Easy Marinara Sauce to each, using the back of a spoon to spread the sauce evenly. Sprinkle a rounded tablespoon of mozzarella over the top of each.

4. Bake until the muffins are nicely toasted and the sauce is heated, about 7 minutes. Turn on the broiler and continue cooking until the cheese begins to brown at bit, 2½ minutes more. Serve immediately.

NOTE

You can add your favorite pizza toppings. Brian loves chopped fried eggplant, while I like to add pepperoncini peppers or olives.

Make sure to not step away once you turn on the broiler since it goes quickly. I have burned many pizza muffins thinking I can multitask!

This is also a fun recipe to let kids help with, adding toppings of their choice.

You can use a toaster oven instead to prepare these.

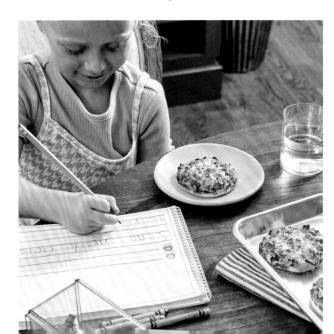

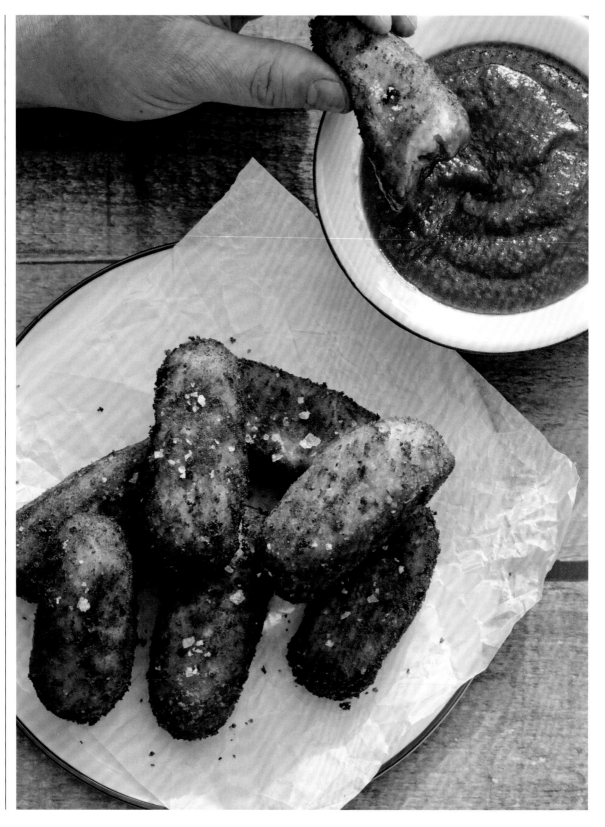

Potato and Bacon Croquettes

MAKES: 1 DOZEN | PREP: 30 MINUTES | COOK: 50 MINUTES | INACTIVE: 25 MINUTES

I was looking through a pile of my grandmother's recipes when I came across this one written on the back of her chicken marsala recipe. I couldn't remember her ever making them, which intrigued me. Measurements were written as "handfuls" and there was no indication of how long she baked them in the oven. After testing her recipe, I eventually added bacon to the mix and found it needed a bit more Parmesan than she had written down. I still have yet to figure out who she made these for or why, but they have since turned into one of Siena's favorite snacks after school.

2¼ pounds (about 4 large) russet potatoes, peeled and cubed (6 cups)

1 tablespoon plus 1 teaspoon kosher salt

3 tablespoons unsalted butter, softened

3 large eggs

½ teaspoon ground black pepper

1 cup shredded low-moisture whole milk mozzarella cheese

¾ cup freshly grated Parmigiano-Reggiano cheese

4 slices thick-cut bacon, cooked and finely chopped

1 cup all-purpose flour plus more for shaping the croquettes

1½ cups Italian-style bread crumbs

1 tablespoon extra-virgin olive oil, plus more for preparing pan

MORE TO SHARE RECIPE

NOTE

When serving the croquettes straight from the oven, I sometimes serve them with a little squeeze of fresh lemon juice.

While rolling the potato croquettes, rinse off your hands every so often to prevent the mixture from sticking to them.

1. Preheat the oven to 400°F. Line a large baking sheet with parchment paper and brush it generously with oil.

2. Put the potatoes in a large pot and add 1 tablespoon of the salt and enough water to cover them. Bring to a boil and cook until fork-tender, about 15 minutes. Drain well and let the potatoes cool for 15 minutes.

3. Transfer the potatoes to a large bowl. Add the butter and mash until smooth. Let cool for 10 minutes more.

4. In a medium bowl, whisk together the eggs, the remaining 1 teaspoon of salt, and the pepper. Add the mozzarella and Parmigiano cheeses and bacon, then mix to combine.

5. Add the egg and cheese mixture to the potatoes and stir until fully mixed. Sprinkle the flour over the top and use a fork to combine.

6. Put the bread crumbs in a shallow bowl. Lightly dust your hands with flour. Using ¼ cup of the potato mixture for each, shape little footballs, then roll them in the bread crumbs, coating completely. Arrange on the prepared baking sheet. When all the croquettes have been shaped, drizzle with oil.

7. Bake until the tops begin to turn golden, about 15 minutes. Carefully turn them and bake until the croquettes are golden brown on all sides, about 20 minutes more. Sprinkle lightly with salt and serve hot. They also can be cooled to room temperature and refrigerated for 3 to 4 days. Reheat at 400°F until warmed through.

Italian Sub~Inspired Stuffed Bread

SERVES: 4 | PREP: 25 MINUTES | COOK: 40 MINUTES | INACTIVE: 1 HOUR

I have great memories of going to the Jersey Shore, and an Italian sub sandwich was my favorite lunch to pack. I almost didn't mind it if I detected some crunchy sand in the mix! This stuffed bread brings me right back to those long afternoons on the beach, where the kids would play together for hours and we'd dodge seagulls when we took out a snack.

1 (1-pound) ball store-bought pizza dough

2 tablespoons red wine vinegar

1 tablespoon extra-virgin olive oil, plus more for preparing the bowl

½ teaspoon dried oregano

½ teaspoon kosher salt

⅛ teaspoon ground black pepper

All-purpose flour, for rolling the dough

4 slices mild or sharp provolone cheese

4 slices deli-sliced mozzarella cheese

6 slices sweet soppressata

6 slices capicola

6 thin slices tomato

5 thin slices red onion

¼ cup sliced pepperoncini

MORE TO SHARE RECIPE

NOTE

You can buy premade pizza dough from your local pizza parlor or find it in the refrigerator section of most grocery stores.

1. Lightly oil the inside of a large bowl. Remove the pizza dough from its packaging and shape it into a ball. Place it in the bowl. Cover and let rise in a warm spot until the dough doubles in size, about 1 hour.

2. Meanwhile, in a small bowl, whisk together the vinegar, oil, oregano, salt, and pepper.

3. Preheat the oven to 375°F. Line a large baking sheet with parchment paper.

4. Lightly flour a work surface. When the dough has doubled in size, punch it down. Roll into a 10 by 12-inch rectangle.

5. Brush the top of the dough with a light coating of the vinegar mixture. Leaving a 1-inch border on the closest 12-inch side, add the provolone cheese, shingling the slices along the length. Repeat with the mozzarella, then the soppressata and, finally, the capicola, stacking them on top of each other. Add the tomatoes and red onion to the top of the capicola, then scatter the pepperoncini over the top. Finish by drizzling 2 teaspoons of the vinegar mixture.

6. Starting at the filled edge, tightly roll the dough like a jelly roll, tucking in the filling, shaping it into a compact log and gently sealing the ends as you go. When you get to the end, press together the dough to seal the roll with a tight seam. Lightly brush the seam with the vinegar mixture, then carefully place the log, seam-side down, on the baking sheet. Working on the baking sheet, tuck in the ends of the log, pinching the dough together to tightly seal. Brush the top of the dough with the remaining vinegar mixture. Using a paring knife, cut three shallow slits across the top of the dough.

7. Bake the loaf until it is cooked through and golden brown, about 40 minutes. Let it rest for 5 to 10 minutes before slicing.

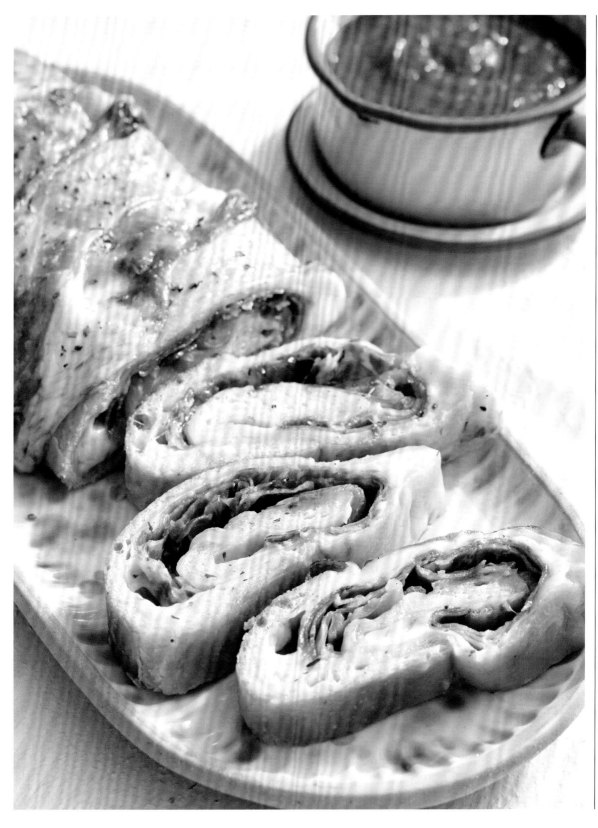

ANOTHER SNACK: LUNCH AND AFTER-SCHOOL WARRIORS

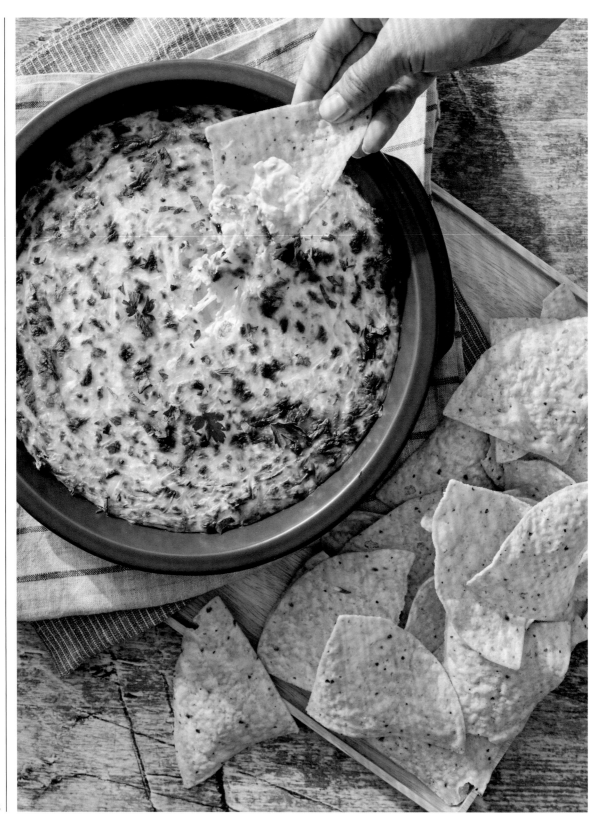

Cherry Pepper Dip

SERVES: 6 TO 8 | PREP: 15 MINUTES | COOK: 25 MINUTES

Be very careful with this recipe—it's the type of dip where you will take just one bite and, next thing you know, more than half of the plate is gone. This dip hits all the right notes: salty, creamy, and a hint of vinegar from the brine, topped off with a bit of honey. My mouth just watered, writing that sentence! Serve it with your favorite type of chips—pita, tortilla, corn, or potato.

1 (8-ounce) package cream cheese, room temperature

½ cup sour cream

¼ cup mayonnaise

1½ teaspoons honey

1 teaspoon hot cherry pepper brine

½ teaspoon kosher salt

¼ teaspoon garlic powder

¼ teaspoon dried oregano

⅛ teaspoon ground black pepper

¾ cup chopped hot cherry peppers

1 cup shredded sharp provolone cheese

1 cup shredded low-moisture whole milk mozzarella cheese

1. Preheat the oven to 375°F.

2. In a medium bowl, mix the cream cheese, sour cream, mayonnaise, honey, cherry pepper brine, salt, garlic powder, oregano, and pepper until smooth and well combined. Fold in the cherry peppers, ½ cup of provolone, and ½ cup of mozzarella.

3. Transfer the mixture to a 9-inch glass baking dish or pie plate, spreading it in a smooth layer. Sprinkle the remaining provolone and mozzarella evenly over the top.

4. Bake until the top begins to get bubbly and the edges start to brown, about 25 minutes. Serve hot.

NOTE

Sometimes you will find seeds in the cherry peppers. Make sure to discard any seeds so they do not make their way into your dip!

Finally, brothers and sisters, whatever is true, whatever is noble, whatever is right, whatever is pure, whatever is lovely, whatever is admirable—if anything is excellent or praiseworthy—think about such things. Whatever you have learned or received or heard from me, or seen in me—put it into practice. And the God of peace will be with you.

PHILIPPIANS 4:8–9

On my worst days of anxiety, I notice that my mind can become my greatest enemy. One thought leads to another, then another, and before I know it I'm lost in a cycle of "should," "maybe," and "what if." Each worry supports the one before with evidence, examples, and conviction.

Satan loves to have you step right up to this merry-go-round and have you believe your circumstances are just as impossible as they seem. Satan wants to feed you lies that center you on "forever" and "never": *You are never going to get better. You are never going to get out of this pit. It will always be like this. You will never grow. You will never progress. You will never repair the relationship. This circumstance will never change.* And on and on the merry-go-round turns.

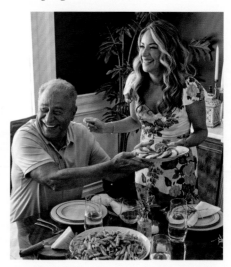

I started to wonder why I invite him into my mind. Some days it's like I pull up a chair, make sure his coffee cup is full, and ask him to stay awhile and tell me all about how he views my situation. Who knows, maybe I even bake him a pie.

Here's the point: I am so ready to accept anxious thoughts, yet when Jesus points me to his promises or asks me to rest in him, I resist. I tell him to come with a PowerPoint presentation, spreadsheets, and a risk assessment, all without so much as asking him if he wants a cup of water. I make sure he doesn't stay past his allotted time, because I have anxiety to tend to.

But what if we're intentional in stopping the merry-go-round? Instead of pouring coffee, we can ask Satan to leave in Jesus's name. I have started gripping the kitchen sink in those moments, praying hard and focusing on these words:

> He said to me, "My grace is sufficient for you, for My strength is made perfect in weakness." . . . Therefore I take pleasure in infirmities, in reproaches, in needs, in persecutions, in distresses, for Christ's sake. For when I am weak, then I am strong.
>
> 2 CORINTHIANS 12:9–10, NKJV

Where we end, he begins. Where we are weak, he is strong. He is not looking for us to pull ourselves out of the anxiety but rather for us to look to him so he can calm the storm and speak peace into our lives. This has taken me years to learn, and I am still working on it. Whenever I feel panic rise and I start proclaiming "forever" and "never," I pray harder.

Dear Lord, when my heart and mind are racing, I pray that I would look to you for peace. That I would lean in to your arms until I feel you wash over me. That my mind would quiet and I would find myself attuned to what you have to say. Help me forsake all other thoughts, surrendering my heart and mind to you.

4

Ahead of the Game: Pre~Prepped Dinners

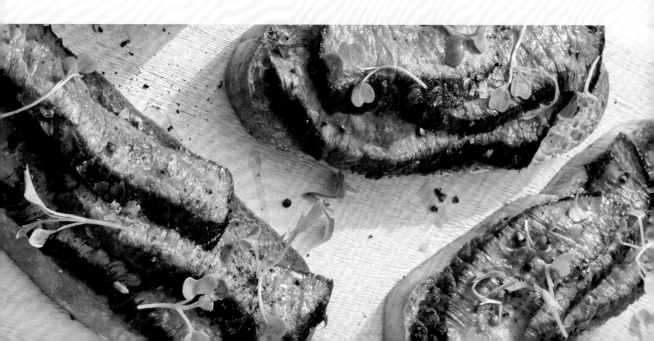

Meal planning and prepping has become an entire lifestyle. What used to be making a simple grocery list before you headed to the store has become a weekly event, with special Tupperware marketed for the purpose and meal-prep subscriptions that will measure out each portion for you.

I used to plan out every meal, Monday through Friday. Now I take an honest look at our week. For those days when time between activities is tight, I give myself a break by planning a slow cooker meal or making it a take-out night. I've also learned that I need to leave room for repurposing meals, reinventing leftovers with deliciously creative uses for them. Most weeks, I end up with more of a three- to four-night plan that keeps me on budget and cuts down on food waste.

Doing this has also helped free me from a bad narrative I had created. I used to feel guilty on nights I couldn't cook dinner, even though no one else was upset. My husband never said a word, but I silently berated myself. If the day or night didn't go according to plan, I would end up cranky, feeling that ordering a pizza was a failure on my part. I wasn't being flexible and I wasn't giving myself grace.

There is a certain sense of satisfaction that comes with having a well-thought-out plan, but life doesn't always go that way. When we include God in our daily plans, we can approach our days with confidence instead of trepidation. He sees our intentions, knows our hearts, and he honors them. He truly does work all things out for good, even if it is not the "good" we had planned.

> All a person's ways seem pure to them,
> but motives are weighed by the LORD.
> Commit to the LORD whatever you do,
> and he will establish your plans.
>
> PROVERBS 16:2–3

Having plans, setting goals, and keeping routines are all good things. But when we find ourselves constantly frustrated, striving, or falling short, maybe it is time to look closely at our plans. Are we leaving room for the inevitable surprises and curveballs? Are we leaving any wiggle room for God's plan?

I didn't plan on having Siena two months early. I didn't plan an emergency C-section or a month in the NICU for her. I didn't plan on struggling through depression, but I also didn't plan on the deliverance that came from these hard times. An increase in my faith led me to share more, which opened doors for a new path in ministry. Likewise, I didn't plan on walking through cancer while writing a book and traveling for conferences. But as I adjusted my expectations and committed to all of this, I realized God's plan was perfect. As I traveled to different states, sharing my testimony and praying for others, an army of women was praying for me.

From the outside, my situation looked challenging, maybe even crazy: juggling multiple deadlines while bracing for scheduled treatments and trying to keep our home life as steady as possible for my daughter. At every point along that road, women from Texas to Orlando laid prayerful hands on me. God was giving me strength that helped me see the beauty of his timing. I was exactly where I needed to be.

> Whoever gives heed to instruction prospers,
> and blessed is the one who trusts in the LORD.
>
> PROVERBS 16:20

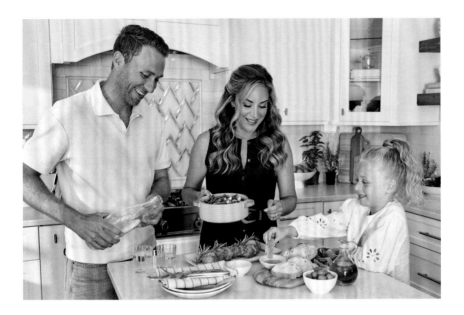

We plan much of our lives: Where will I go to college? What career path will I take? Who will I marry, and where will we live? We also face mundane choices, such as what to wear and what to eat for lunch. And, *do I really need that candle from Target?* Interruptions in our plans do not have to be total losses. They can be a necessary redirection or can lead to opportunities we wouldn't otherwise consider.

Think of the disciples. Most of them had other plans for their lives. Andrew, Peter, John, and James had intended to be fishermen. In Matthew 4, they were about to cast nets in the sea when Jesus said, "Come, follow me" (v. 19). No doubt this led them on a greater journey than they could have imagined for themselves. Why not leave room in our planning for God's great diversion?

Dear Lord, please help me continually surrender to you. To include you in all decisions big and small. To trust in your timing and your plan. Help me not be stubborn in my ways. Help me not to be prideful and rooted in my own ways. Give me a heart that yields to your direction and correction, knowing that I will find great joy and contentment in the plans you have for me.

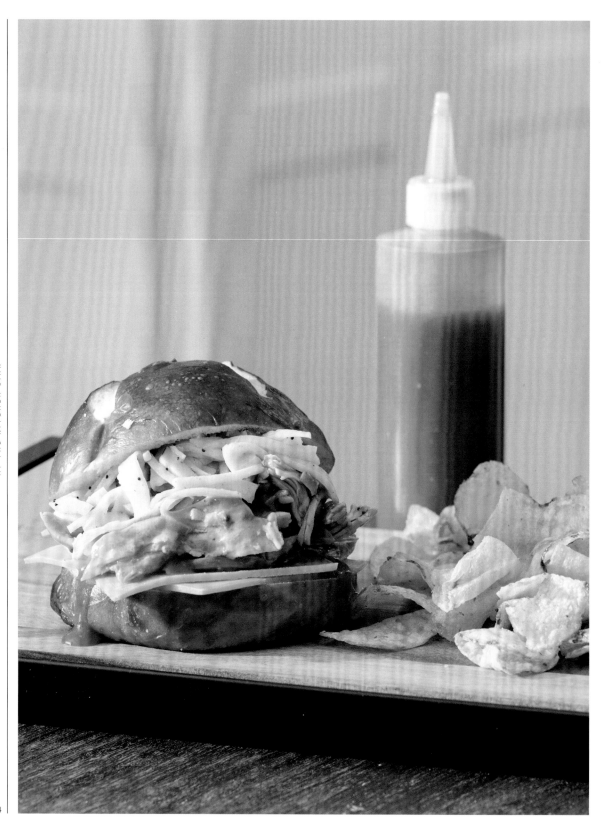

Apple Cider Chicken Sandwiches

There are many reasons this is a perfect dish for the fall season. For starters, it's a great way to use the apple cider you keep grabbing from the farm stand or grocery store. You can set this up in a slow cooker, and it'll be done by the time you get home from the football field. It's just an all-around feel-good recipe for the season!

1½ cups apple cider

½ cup packed light brown sugar

1 tablespoon whole-grain mustard

1½ teaspoons chipotle hot sauce

1 teaspoon Worcestershire sauce

1 teaspoon kosher salt

½ teaspoon paprika

½ teaspoon ground black pepper

2 pounds boneless, skinless chicken breasts

½ yellow onion, sliced in ½-inch-thick half moons

1 cup ketchup

1 tablespoon cornstarch

6 slices Cheddar cheese

6 pretzel buns or rolls of your choice

Apple Fennel Slaw, for serving (page 89)

NOTE

You will most likely have some sauce left over. Refrigerate it in an airtight container, using it for sandwiches during the week.

Leftover braising liquid that's not used in the sauce can be refrigerated or frozen. Use it for another batch of the sauce, if desired. Bring to a full boil for 5 minutes before proceeding with the recipe.

1. In the base of a slow cooker, whisk together the apple cider, brown sugar, mustard, hot sauce, Worcestershire sauce, salt, paprika, and pepper. Add the chicken and onions, layering them evenly and coating with the braising liquid.

2. Cover and cook on low until the chicken is fork-tender, about 5 hours.

3. Using tongs, remove the chicken from the cooking liquid and transfer it to a medium bowl. Strain the cooking liquid through a fine mesh strainer into a small saucepan; reserve 1 cup to use for the recipe. Any excess can be refrigerated, if desired (see Note).

4. Add the ketchup to the strained liquid, stirring to combine. Place over medium heat.

5. Stir together the cornstarch and 3 tablespoons of cold water to make a slurry, then whisk it into the saucepan. Bring to a simmer and cook, stirring frequently, until the mixture thickens, 8 to 10 minutes.

6. Meanwhile, working right in the bowl, use two forks to shred the chicken. Add ¾ cup of the thickened sauce and toss to coat.

7. To assemble the sandwiches, place a slice of cheese on the bottom half of each bun and add about ½ cup of shredded chicken. Top with the Apple Fennel Slaw and add the top bun.

Veggie~Packed Fresh Salmon Cakes

MAKES: 32 PATTIES | PREP: 30 MINUTES | COOK: 1 HOUR | INACTIVE: 30 MINUTES

When Siena was first getting into solid foods, pretty much anything in patty form was a win. These were born out of a desire to have something that we all could enjoy at dinnertime. Plus, I was trying to get as many veggies in her as I could! These are still a family dinner favorite. You can customize them by playing with the veggies, adapting them to your preference and what's on hand.

FOR THE SAUCE

½ cup mayonnaise

2 tablespoons sweet relish

1 tablespoon ketchup

2 teaspoons freshly squeezed lemon juice

½ teaspoon salt

¼ teaspoon ground black pepper

FOR THE SALMON CAKES

1 (1-pound) salmon fillet

1½ teaspoons extra-virgin olive oil

1½ teaspoons kosher salt

½ teaspoon ground black pepper

3 tablespoons coconut oil

¼ cup chopped red onion

1 tablespoon chopped garlic

1 tablespoon capers, drained and coarsely chopped

1 cup frozen riced broccoli, thawed

1 cup baby-cut carrots, minced

2 tablespoons Dijon mustard

1 tablespoon honey

1½ teaspoons Old Bay seasoning

1 teaspoon soy sauce

1 cup panko bread crumbs

2 large eggs, beaten

Lemon wedges, for serving

1. **MAKE THE SAUCE:** In a small bowl, whisk together the mayonnaise, relish, ketchup, lemon juice, salt, and pepper. Refrigerate until ready to use.

2. **MAKE THE SALMON CAKES:** Preheat the oven to 375°F. Line a baking sheet with parchment paper.

3. Place the salmon skin-side down on the baking sheet. Drizzle with olive oil and season with ¼ teaspoon each of the salt and the pepper.

4. Bake until the thickest part of the fillet registers 145°F, 12 to 15 minutes. Let cool completely.

5. Meanwhile, in a large sauté pan over medium heat, warm 1 tablespoon of the coconut oil. Add the onion, garlic, and capers. Cook, stirring frequently, until fragrant, 1 minute. Add the riced broccoli, carrots, ½ teaspoon of the salt, and ¼ teaspoon of the pepper. Continue cooking, stirring often, until the vegetables have somewhat softened, 5 to 6 minutes.

6. Transfer the vegetables to a large bowl and cool completely. When they are cool, add the mustard, honey, Old Bay, and soy sauce and mix well.

7. Remove and discard the skin from the salmon. Using your hands, flake the salmon into small pieces, adding them to the vegetable mixture along with the panko and eggs. Fold lightly to combine.

8. Line a large baking sheet with parchment paper.

9. Using a 1-ounce (2 tablespoons) cookie scoop, portion the salmon mixture into mounds and place on the baking sheet. With your hands, shape the mounds into 2½-inch

CONTINUED ON PAGE 88

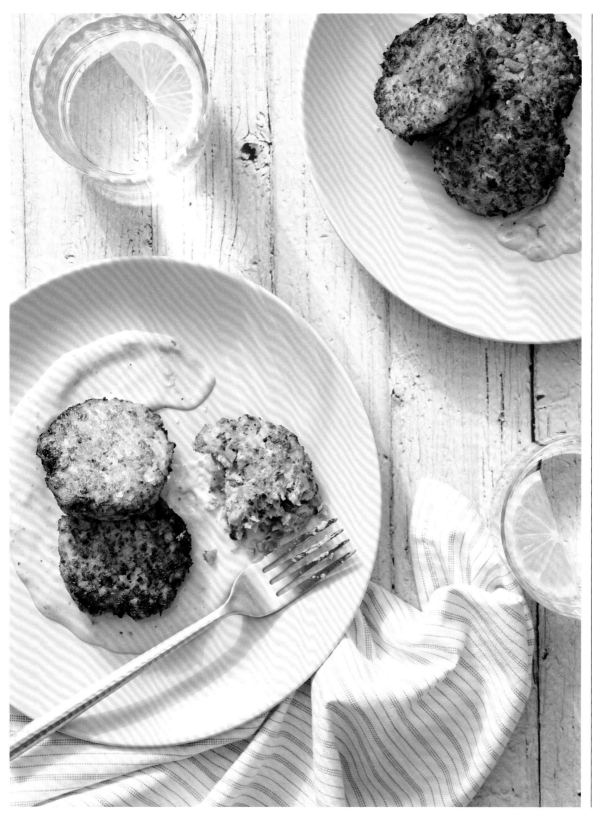

A HEAD OF THE GAME: PRE-PREPPED DINNERS

patties about ½-inch thick. Cover the pan with plastic wrap and refrigerate at least 30 minutes before cooking.

10. Using the same sauté pan over medium heat, warm 1 tablespoon of the coconut oil. Working in batches, cook the patties, turning once, until nicely browned on each side, 6 to 7 minutes per side. After they're cooked, transfer the patties to a paper towel–lined plate. Add more oil as needed and continue cooking.

11. To serve, spoon about 1 tablespoon of the sauce onto a serving plate, making a swoosh with the back of a spoon, if desired. Top with two to four patties and serve with a lemon wedge.

NOTE

You can use a food processor to finely chop the carrots.

If you can't find riced broccoli in the store, it is easy to make. For a quick how-to, see the Note with the recipe for Crispy Broccoli and Cheese Rice Balls (page 70).

Apple Fennel Slaw

SERVES: 6 | PREP: 15 MINUTES | INACTIVE: 1 HOUR 30 MINUTES

The crispy combination of fennel and apple is not to be missed, the sweetness of the apples complementing the subtle licorice flavor of the fennel. Make sure not to skip the first step. Salting the fennel and drawing out excess liquid helps keep the slaw crisp.

2 small fennel bulbs, thinly sliced

2½ teaspoons kosher salt

1 large Gala apple, julienned

¼ cup extra-virgin olive oil

2 tablespoons apple cider vinegar

1 tablespoon mayonnaise

¼ teaspoon honey

½ teaspoon poppy seeds

⅛ teaspoon ground mustard

½ teaspoon celery salt

⅛ teaspoon ground black pepper

1. Place the fennel in a large colander, sprinkle 1½ teaspoons of the salt over the fennel, and gently toss to distribute. Let it sit for 30 minutes to draw out excess water. Shake off any excess liquid and, using paper towels, dry the fennel, gently pressing to release excess water.

2. Transfer to a large bowl. Add the apples and toss to combine.

3. In a small bowl, vigorously whisk the oil, apple cider vinegar, mayonnaise, honey, poppy seeds, ground mustard, celery salt, pepper, and the remaining 1 teaspoon of kosher salt until emulsified.

4. Pour the mixture over the fennel and apples and toss to coat. Cover and place in the refrigerator for 1 hour. Toss once more before serving.

NOTE

I use a mandoline set at the ⅛-inch mark to slice the fennel. You can also use a sharp knife and slice as thin as possible.

This pairs well with the Apple Cider Chicken Sandwiches (page 85).

The sweetness of the apples with the crunchy fennel makes for a light slaw to use as a side or to top your sandwiches. I also love eating a big bowl of it for lunch and maybe throwing a couple of pieces of grilled chicken on top.

When we think of heroes in the Bible, many of us would cite Moses, Paul, David, and Daniel. Maybe even Esther or Mary. However, as I finished reading the book of Job, I found myself praying, *God give me a relentless faith like that of Job.*

At the beginning of the book, we get a small glimpse into the man's life, his thriving household, and his family. Then Satan comes to God, questioning the true depth of Job's faith.

> **The LORD said to Satan, "Have you considered my servant Job? There is no one on earth like him; he is blameless and upright, a man who fears God and shuns evil."**
>
> JOB 1:8

Satan then challenges God, saying, in my paraphrase, "Of course Job worships you, his life is great! Let me start ruining things for him and see if he is still praising you!" As the story goes, Satan sets out to destroy Job and all that he has, leaving him in a state of utter ruin to prove his point. We can get into debates and question why God allowed this. But the last time I read the story, I had a new view: God thought so highly of Job that he allowed Satan to test him. Imagine God knowing that your faith and your love for him are strong enough that he can use you in this manner. How amazing to be the one that Jesus uses to prove the devil wrong!

Job's life was interrupted. His circumstances kept changing, and he wasn't sure why. But in the face of these trials, he was committed to laying himself at the feet of God. He trusted the Lord even without understanding what was happening to him.

We often try to find explanations for our suffering, but they are beyond us. We live in a sinful and fallen world, yet we know that he has overcome the world and is never out of reach. Job knew that God was his protector, even when it felt as if everything was against him. His friends pointed out how he may be wrong, and his wife essentially said he was crazy, yet Job stood firm, tightening his grip on the Lord's hand.

But He knows the way I take;
When He has put me to the test, I will come out as gold.
My foot has held on to His path;
I have kept His way and not turned aside.

Job's patience and faith endured in the end. He accepted God's plan even though he didn't understand it. Just as an athlete needs to practice to get stronger, so do we. God wastes nothing. Our progress, those small steps of obedience, our relentless faith—all of that scares the devil. He would have you believe your faith and obedience are worthless when they are worth everything.

Where do you need to be more relentless in your faith today?

―――――――――――

Dear Lord, please help me be just as relentless as Job. Help me not grow weary in reaching for your hand. Although I may be exasperated or exhausted by circumstances, help me cling to you as the storm rages. While I may not understand every-thing, allow me to remain confident that you are in control of situations that seem out of control. Help me to build upon my faith for the long run.

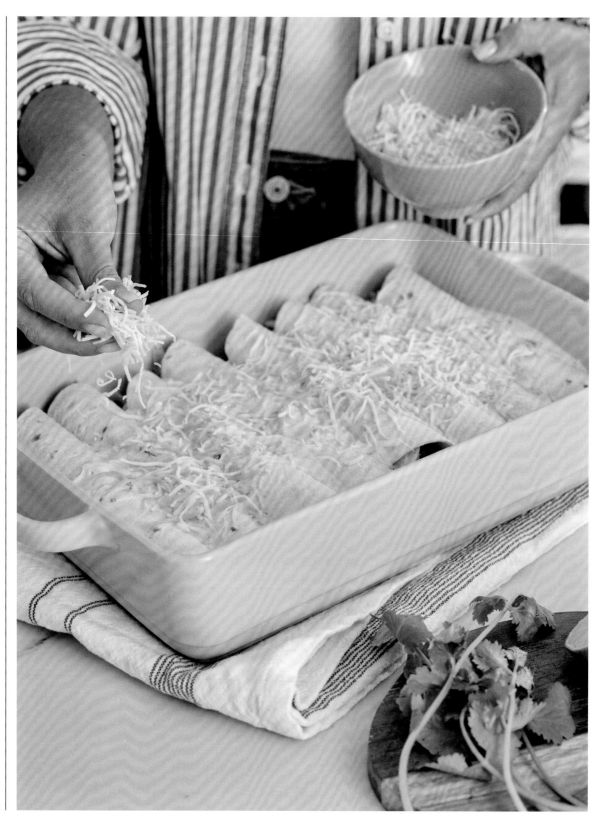

Rotisserie Chicken Avocado Enchiladas

SERVES: 6 | PREP: 20 MINUTES | COOK: 35 MINUTES

Baked in a creamy sauce that's laced with salsa verde, these enchiladas have a different vibe than traditional red-sauced versions. They're also another chance for rotisserie chicken to be an easy meal prep hero. This dish is a welcome addition to our Sunday dinner lineup. Even my dad agrees to deviate from Sunday gravy when they're on the menu.

1 tablespoon unsalted butter

1 tablespoon minced garlic

1½ teaspoons all-purpose flour

1 cup chicken broth

Juice of ½ lime

1 teaspoon ground cumin

1 teaspoon kosher salt

¼ teaspoon onion powder

¼ teaspoon chipotle chili powder

⅛ teaspoon ground black pepper

½ cup mild salsa verde

½ cup sour cream

¼ cup chopped fresh cilantro, plus more for serving

8 (8-inch) flour tortillas

2 cups shredded rotisserie chicken

2 small avocados, thinly sliced

2 cups finely shredded Mexican blend cheese

Hot sauce, for serving

Lime wedges, for serving

1. Preheat the oven to 375°F.

2. In a large sauté pan over medium heat, melt the butter. Add the garlic and cook, stirring several times, until fragrant, about 1 minute. Stir in the flour and cook until it is lightly colored, 1 minute.

3. Whisk in the chicken broth and bring to a simmer. Cook, stirring several times, until slightly thickened, about 2 minutes.

4. Whisk in the lime juice, cumin, salt, onion powder, chili powder, and pepper and remove from the heat. Stir in the salsa verde, sour cream, and cilantro.

5. In a 9 by 13-inch baking dish, spread ½ cup of the sauce over the bottom.

6. Place a tortilla on a flat work surface and add ¼ cup of the chicken filling off center and toward one side. Top with 3 slices of avocado and 1 tablespoon of the cheese. Roll in a tight tube and place seam-side down, in the baking dish. Continue filling and rolling the tortillas. When all have been added to the baking dish, spoon the remaining sauce over the top and sprinkle with the remaining cheese.

7. Bake, uncovered, until the filling is hot all the way through and the cheese is melted, about 30 minutes. Serve immediately with cilantro, hot sauce, and lime wedges.

MORE TO SHARE RECIPE

Rotisserie Chicken Spinach Stuffed Shells

SERVES: 6 TO 8 | PREP: 30 MINUTES | COOK: 1 HOUR

Adding the rotisserie chicken to these stuffed shells serves two purposes: It makes the meal a bit heartier, and it also serves as a shortcut. I like to prep this dish the night before or first thing in the morning. That way I can just pop it in the oven after a busy day or when our company arrives. It is also one of my favorite dishes to drop off to a neighbor or friend in need of a meal.

FOR THE SHELLS

1 tablespoon plus 1 teaspoon kosher salt

24 jumbo pasta shells

2 cups chopped rotisserie chicken

1 cup whole milk ricotta cheese

1 cup chopped fresh baby spinach

½ cup low-moisture whole milk shredded mozzarella cheese

1 large egg, lightly beaten

1 teaspoon lemon zest

½ teaspoon ground black pepper

FOR THE SAUCE

6 tablespoons unsalted butter

3 tablespoons chopped garlic

3 tablespoons all-purpose flour

1 cup dry white wine

1½ cups whole milk, warmed

1¼ cups shredded low-moisture whole milk mozzarella

¾ cup plus 2 tablespoons freshly grated Parmigiano-Reggiano cheese

salt and ground black pepper

MORE TO SHARE RECIPE

1. Preheat the oven to 375°F.

2. **MAKE THE SHELLS:** Bring a large pot of water to a boil and add 1 tablespoon of the salt. Add the shells and cook, stirring often, until al dente, 8 to 9 minutes. Drain, reserving ½ cup of the cooking water for the sauce.

3. In a large bowl, mix the chicken, ricotta, spinach, mozzarella, egg, lemon zest, remaining 1 teaspoon of salt, and the pepper until well combined. Fill the pasta shells, using 1 heaping tablespoon of the chicken mixture for each. Arrange on a large plate or baking sheet and set aside.

4. **MAKE THE SAUCE:** In a large saucepan over medium-low heat, melt the butter. Add the garlic and cook, stirring several times, until fragrant, 30 to 40 seconds. Stir in the flour. Cook, stirring several times, until it starts to bubble and color very slightly, 1 minute.

5. Whisking constantly as you do so, slowly add the wine and then bring the mixture to a simmer. Slowly whisk in the milk and bring the mixture to a gentle simmer, stirring often. Cook until it has thickened enough to coat the back of a spoon, 2 to 3 minutes.

6. Remove the pan from heat and stir in ¾ cup each of the mozzarella and Parmigiano cheeses, the salt, and pepper.

7. Spread ¾ cup of the sauce over the bottom of a 9 by 13-inch baking dish, then arrange the shells filling-side up. To the remaining sauce in the pan, stir in the ½ cup reserved pasta cooking water. Spoon the sauce evenly over the shells and sprinkle with the remaining ½ cup of mozzarella and 2 tablespoons of Parmigiano.

8. Cover the pan with aluminum foil and bake for 20 minutes. Uncover and continue baking until the top is bubbly, 18 to 20 minutes more. Let sit for 3 to 4 minutes before serving.

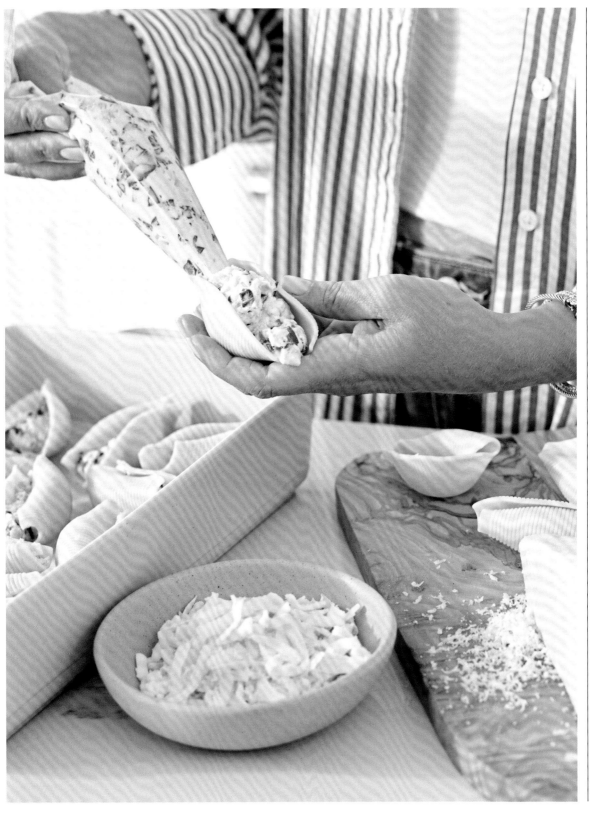

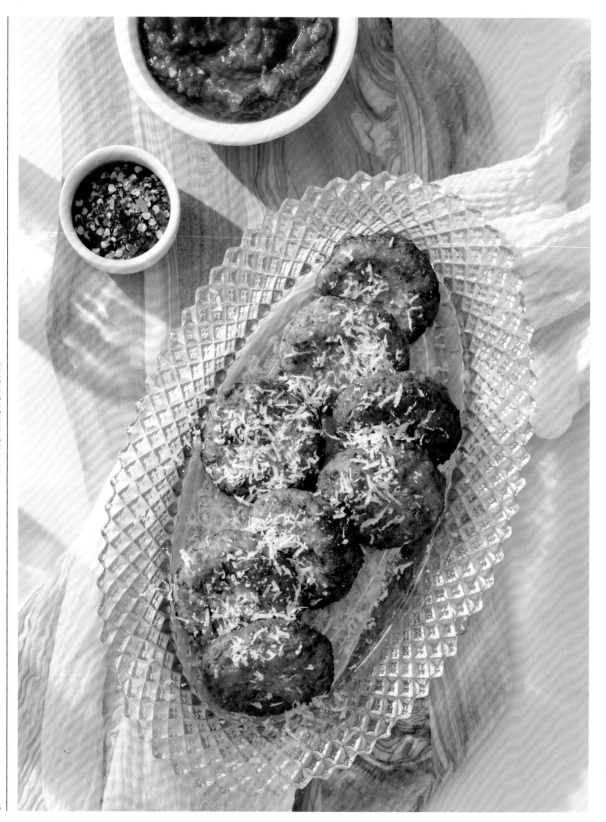

Crispy Chickpea Fritters
with Spicy Marinara

SERVES: 4 | PREP: 15 MINUTES | COOK: 35 MINUTES

I will be honest: I created these fritters so I could have an excuse to make the spicy marinara! But I'll also make them when I am doing a choose-your-adventure type of night. I put out a large platter with chunks of feta, store-bought grape leaves, triangles of pita, some chopped salad, and tzatziki sauce. Everyone makes their own plate, and everyone is happy!

FOR THE SPICY MARINARA

2 tablespoons extra-virgin olive oil

1 small yellow onion, chopped

3 large garlic cloves

1 to 2 tablespoons hot cherry pepper brine

1½ tablespoons unsalted butter

½ teaspoon crushed red pepper flakes

¼ teaspoon sugar

1 (28-ounce) can crushed tomatoes

1 teaspoon dried basil

Kosher salt

FOR THE FRITTERS

1 (15-ounce) can chickpeas, drained and rinsed

⅓ cup fresh parsley leaves

¼ cup finely grated pecorino Romano cheese, plus more for serving

3 cloves garlic, chopped

1½ teaspoons capers, drained

1 teaspoon lemon zest

Kosher salt

Ground black pepper

1 large egg

3 tablespoons all-purpose flour

Extra-virgin olive oil, for pan frying

MORE TO SHARE RECIPE

1. **MAKE THE MARINARA:** In a medium skillet, warm the oil over medium-high heat. Add the onion and garlic and cook, stirring often, until the onions are translucent and begin to take on the slightest bit of color, 5 to 7 minutes. Add the cherry pepper brine, butter, red pepper flakes, and sugar, stirring until the butter melts.

2. Stir in the crushed tomatoes and basil and bring to a simmer. Cook, stirring often until slightly thickened, about 15 minutes. Add salt to taste. The sauce can be made in advance and refrigerated in a tightly sealed container for up to 3 days or frozen.

3. Meanwhile, **MAKE THE FRITTERS:** In a food processor fitted with the S blade, pulse together the chickpeas, parsley, cheese, garlic, capers, lemon zest, and a generous pinch of salt and pepper until uniformly chopped but still chunky. Do not puree.

4. Transfer the chickpea mixture to a large bowl and add the egg and flour. Stir to combine.

5. With lightly moistened hands, shape the mixture into eight equal-size patties.

6. In a large nonstick skillet over medium-high heat, warm ½ inch of oil. When it is hot, add the patties in batches. Cook, turning once, until they are golden brown, about 3 minutes per side. Transfer to a paper towel–lined plate.

7. Serve warm with the Spicy Marinara and a sprinkling of pecorino cheese.

NOTE

These fritters also make a great option for your kiddo's lunch box!

Not Your Average Sloppy Joe

SERVES: 6 | PREP: 15 MINUTES | COOK: 15 MINUTES | INACTIVE: 4 HOURS

Full disclosure: I used to strongly dislike when my mom had sloppy joes on the menu. My mom is a great cook, but she has a weak spot for a meat sauce that comes in a can. Let's not even talk about Spam, or canned peas as a side. I'm sorry, Mom! I knew there had to be a better way, and this recipe is it! These sloppy joes are kid-tested and approved by my daughter and nieces, along with the adults in tow.

1 tablespoon extra-virgin olive oil

2 garlic cloves, finely chopped

½ cup chopped onion

1 large red bell pepper, diced

1 tablespoon balsamic vinegar

1 cup ketchup

¼ cup apple cider vinegar

¼ cup packed light brown sugar

3 tablespoons Worcestershire sauce

1 tablespoon Dijon mustard

1½ teaspoons chipotle chili powder

1 teaspoon kosher salt, plus more as needed

½ teaspoon ground black pepper, plus more as needed

1 pound ground turkey (93% lean)

1 tablespoon cornstarch

6 slices muenster cheese

6 potato buns

1. In a large skillet over medium heat, warm the oil. Add the garlic and cook, stirring several times, until fragrant, 30 seconds. Add the onions and cook until they begin to soften, 2 minutes. Stir in the red pepper and balsamic vinegar. Cook, stirring occasionally, until all the vegetables are soft, 4 to 5 minutes.

2. Meanwhile, in a slow cooker, stir together the ketchup, apple cider vinegar, brown sugar, Worcestershire sauce, mustard, chili powder, salt, and pepper.

3. When the vegetables are soft, add them to the slow cooker and return the skillet to medium heat. Add the turkey to the skillet and cook, stirring and crumbling the meat, until no pink remains, 6 to 7 minutes. Add salt and pepper to taste and add the turkey to the slow cooker.

4. Cover the slow cooker and cook on high for 3½ hours.

5. In a small bowl, make a slurry with the cornstarch and 1 tablespoon of cold water. Stir the mixture into the slow cooker and turn the heat to high. Cook until the sauce thickens, about 20 minutes more.

6. To serve, place a slice of the cheese on the bottom half of each bun, add a generous scoop of the turkey mixture, and top with the bun.

NOTE

I love serving this with half sour pickles and coleslaw on the side.

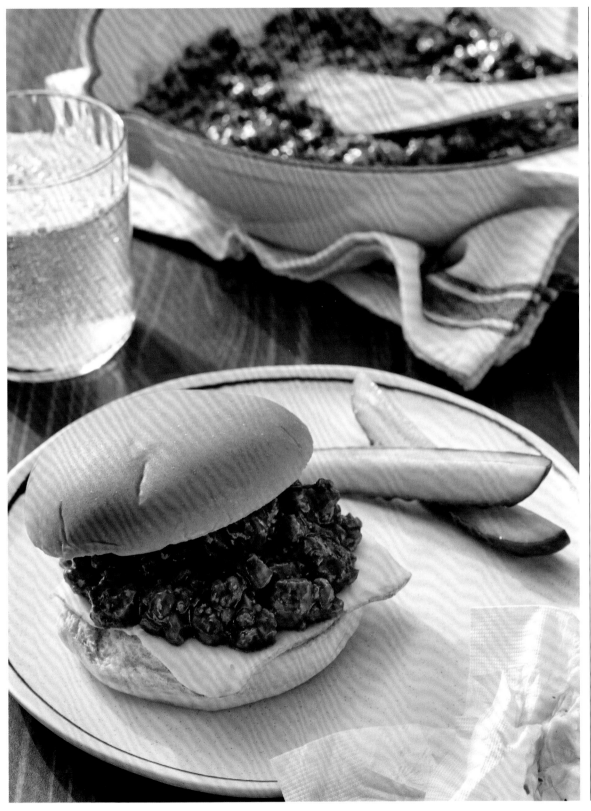

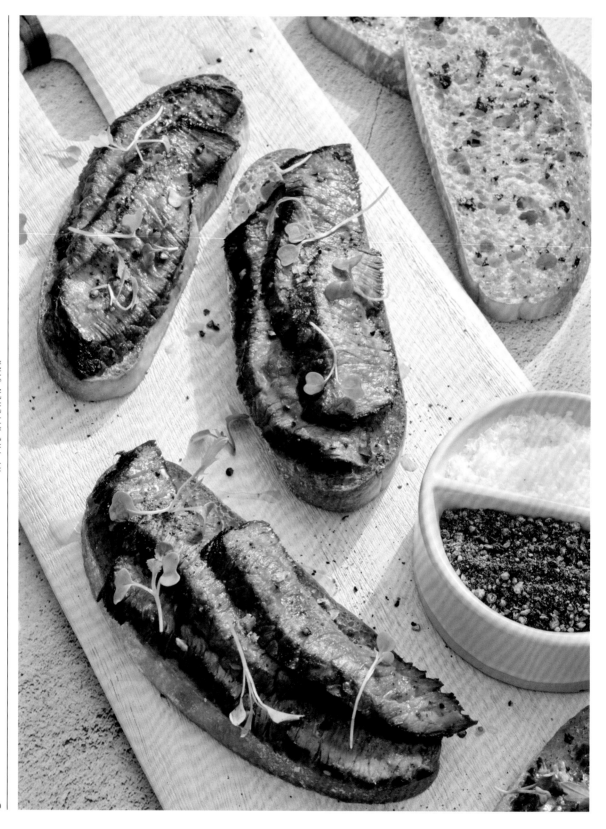

London Broil Toast

SERVES: 6 | PREP: 15 MINUTES | COOK: 15 MINUTES | INACTIVE: 1 HOUR 30 MINUTES

On the Fourth of July, the main event was not the fireworks. Rather it was afterward, when my uncle would serve these pieces of London broil on top of slices of Italian bread. We looked forward to it every year!

FOR THE STEAK

1 (1½ pounds) London broil

¼ cup extra-virgin olive oil

3 tablespoons light brown sugar

2 tablespoons soy sauce

1½ tablespoons chopped garlic

1 tablespoon Worcestershire sauce

½ teaspoon kosher salt

¼ teaspoon ground black pepper

2 tablespoons unsalted butter, plus more, as needed

2 sprigs fresh rosemary

Flaky sea salt, for serving

FOR THE TOAST

4 tablespoons (½ stick) unsalted butter, melted

1½ teaspoons chopped fresh parsley

1 teaspoon minced garlic

6 thick slices crusty bread

Kosher salt

Ground black pepper

NOTE

Add greens by layering fresh baby spinach or arugula on top of the bread, then the London broil.

The term *London broil* usually refers to a cooking method with a thick cut of beef. Traditionally, a flank steak or top round cut would be used for this recipe.

1. **MAKE THE STEAK:** Place the meat in a large ziplock bag.

2. In a small bowl, mix the oil, brown sugar, soy sauce, garlic, Worcestershire sauce, salt, and pepper until the sugar dissolves. Pour over the meat, seal the bag, and turn it over several times so it is well coated. Refrigerate for at least 1 hour or overnight. Remove from the refrigerator 20 minutes before cooking.

3. Place a large cast-iron skillet over medium heat. Add the butter and let it melt and sizzle. Meanwhile, use tongs to remove the steak from the marinade, letting the excess drip off, then gently blot the meat dry with paper towels. Add the meat to the hot skillet and cook, without turning, until well browned on the bottom, 4 to 5 minutes. Flip the steak and place the rosemary sprigs around the meat. If the pan seems dry, add a pat of butter. Cook until the internal temperature of the meat registers 135°F for medium-rare, 4 to 6 minutes, depending on the thickness of the meat; it will continue to rise a few degrees when it is removed from the heat. Transfer to a cutting board, tent with aluminum foil, and let rest for 10 minutes.

4. **MAKE THE TOAST:** While the meat is resting, turn on the broiler and line a baking sheet with parchment paper.

5. In a small bowl, combine the melted butter, parsley, and garlic. Arrange the bread slices on the baking sheet, brush with the butter mixture, and sprinkle with salt and pepper.

6. Just before broiling the toast, cut the meat, across the grain, into thin slices. Cover with foil. Place the toasts under the broiler. Watching closely, broil until the bread is golden brown, 1 to 2 minutes.

7. To serve, top each piece of toast with 3 to 4 slices of meat, drizzle lightly with pan drippings and sprinkle with flaky sea salt.

5

Carpool Cuisine: Weeknight Eat and Go

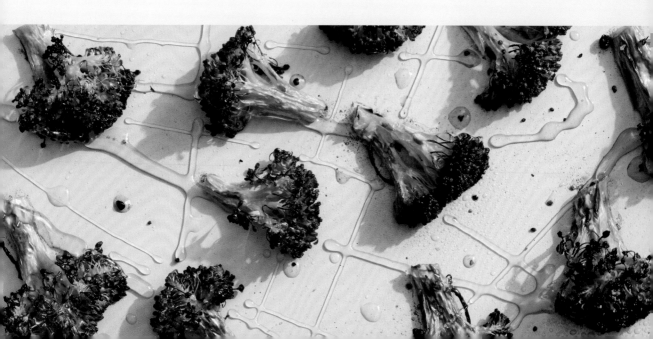

et's face it, at times our lives feel like we are running Fortune 500 companies—without the vacation days and corner offices. We're managing homes, careers, social lives, extracurriculars, and church activities—often for multiple people—and our to-do lists can feel relentless. Most nights, we fall asleep counting things still needing to be done instead of sheep.

Having your go-to recipes for nights when there isn't much time to think or cook can eliminate a lot of trips to the drive-thru. They're recipes that become sort of like reflexes. Roasted Broccoli with Honey (page 120) appears on Siena's plate two or three times a week, while Easy Marinara Sauce (page 111) is a springboard for many simple dishes, including all kinds of pasta. And you can always rely on the Chicken Cutlet Sandwiches (page 108) or the Smoky Sweet Potato and Farro Bowl (page 107) in between sports practices.

Amid the day-to-day chaos, God wants us to take hold of him. Sometimes we need to take inventory of our lives and examine our priorities. When we allow for this, he can help bear our burdens and soothe our hurried, anxious hearts.

Although I'm an experienced home cook, I still make mistakes in the kitchen. I have messed up boxed cake mixes, burned plenty of garlic bread, and had sauces come out looking like glue. And at least every other time I make rice, the pot ends up boiling over or burning, leaving me with a messy pan to scrub.

In life, too, I am guilty of letting things simmer. I try my best to adjust the flame every so often so I do not boil over. Life happens, though, and I am human. Usually it starts with me ignoring something small, like the fact that I'm the only one picking up things off the stairs, or it's the third morning in a row that Siena has refused to wear the clothes we picked out the night before. Someone asks, "Why are you so grumpy?" Then, *boom!* The explosion of emotions happens, and the fallout hits everyone. In its wake, I am left with a whole bunch of shame, guilt, and disappointment that needs to be cleaned up.

So many of us end up in that place over and over, especially when we harbor guilt or feelings of inadequacy. Sometimes we even feel justified in our boil over. How much can one person be expected to take?

> Hear my cry, O God; listen to my prayer.
>
> From the end of the earth will I cry to You, when my heart is overwhelmed and fainting; lead me to the rock that is higher than I [yes, a rock that is too high for me].
>
> For You have been a shelter and a refuge for me, a strong tower against the adversary.
>
> I will dwell in Your tabernacle forever; let me find refuge and trust in the shelter of Your wings. Selah [pause, and calmly and think of that]!
>
> PSALM 61:1–4, AMPC

Keeping everything at a simmer uses more energy than we know. Have you ever just cried out to God? Maybe you have gripped the kitchen sink with your head down, and asked, *Why?* Or maybe you have sat, head in hands, feeling that you had reached capacity. We do not need to come to

God put together, with our thoughts neatly organized. Our prayers don't need to be carefully packaged or full of restraint. He wants us to be vulnerable, open, and honest with him. We should feel safe to let it all out at his feet. What better place than in the presence of the one who can bear it all?

I love how Psalm 61 instructs us to pause and "calmly think of that." Find refuge and strength in Jesus, and then take a minute to let his peace wash over you as you wait in his presence. He hears you, and he sees how overwhelmed you are feeling. Let him slow down your racing thoughts. Petition him for clearheaded thinking and God-given solutions to whatever causes you to reach your breaking point. Allow him room to reveal the solutions. Maybe it's you being more honest with your husband about the help you need. Maybe it's taking deep breaths instead of going off the deep end after a surprise email from a client. Or maybe it's taking a short break before jumping to the next assignment or activity.

If only life was made up of perfectly orchestrated and harmonious moments. It isn't, though. Knowing that we don't have to bring prayers to God in an organized, controlled fashion can be a huge weight from our shoulders. We can simply ugly cry at his feet. He promises that, in our time of need, he will hear us and offer strength and refuge—and possibly the gentle reminder that it's okay to order pizza tonight.

Dear Lord, please grant peace to my troubled heart and mind. Hear my cry of frustration when I feel lost within the storm. Remind me that you are my strong tower and my shelter and that I can renew my strength in you. Provide a way where there seems to be no way. Help me see the path forward. Give me the words to convey my needs and accept help from those who can come alongside me. Help me to reset if needed and rest in you.

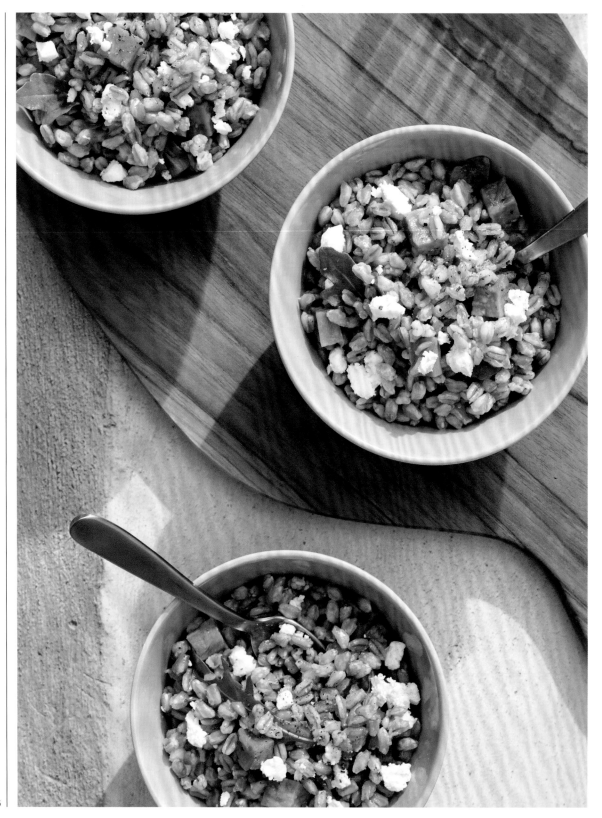

Smoky Sweet Potato and Farro Bowl

SERVES: 6 | PREP: 20 MINUTES | COOK: 35 MINUTES

I love using farro as a base for a bowl. You can get creative and top it with almost anything. For this recipe, the sweet potatoes become caramelized in the oven, which is my favorite part. The smoked paprika is a key ingredient; a little bit goes a long way. Paired with goat cheese and maple vinaigrette, it is great for a light dinner. Or store in an airtight container, undressed, and have it for lunch the next couple of days!

FOR THE POTATOES

2 medium sweet potatoes, peeled and cubed (about 3 cups)

2 tablespoons extra-virgin olive oil

1 tablespoon light brown sugar

1 teaspoon kosher salt

½ teaspoon smoked paprika

¼ teaspoon ground black pepper

2 cups farro

1 (8-ounce) container crumbled goat cheese

3 cups baby arugula

FOR THE VINAIGRETTE

½ cup extra-virgin olive oil

2 tablespoons maple syrup

1½ tablespoons rice vinegar

1 tablespoon freshly squeezed orange juice

1½ teaspoons finely chopped shallot

1½ teaspoons chopped fresh tarragon (or 1 teaspoon dried tarragon)

MORE TO SHARE RECIPE

1. **MAKE THE POTATOES:** Preheat the oven to 425°F.

2. Scatter the sweet potatoes on a large rimmed baking sheet. Drizzle the oil over the top and season with the brown sugar, salt, smoked paprika, and pepper; toss to combine.

3. Bake, tossing once halfway through, until the sweet potatoes are fork-tender and begin to brown on the edges, 30 to 35 minutes.

4. Meanwhile, cook the farro according to the package directions; set aside.

5. **MAKE THE VINAIGRETTE:** In a small bowl, whisk together the oil, maple syrup, vinegar, orange juice, shallots, and tarragon until well combined and emulsified.

6. In a large bowl, gently toss together the sweet potatoes, farro, and vinaigrette.

7. Transfer to a large serving platter and sprinkle the goat cheese evenly over the farro. Serve with a heap of arugula piled on top of the bowl.

NOTE

A drizzle of olive oil, a sprinkling of orange zest, and a handful of dried cranberries or nuts are among the many ways the bowls can be customized.

Farro absorbs a lot of the vinaigrette and especially the seasonings, so taste and adjust as necessary before serving. If you don't plan on serving it right away, add the vinaigrette and toss right before serving.

Alternatively, you can toss the goat cheese and arugula with the farro. The goat cheese will melt into the farro and add a creaminess, while the arugula will wilt, but it's delicious!

Chicken Cutlet Sandwiches
with Roasted Red Pepper Mayo

SERVES: 4 | PREP: 15 MINUTES | COOK: 10 MINUTES

Being able to make a good chicken cutlet is a necessary kitchen skill in my book. I have distinct memories of my grandmother serving up hot, crispy cutlets right from the pan, always paired with a sliced tomato salad. A freshly made chicken cutlet can be a base for a delicious sandwich, or can turn into a fancy Milanese when you top it with arugula. I am pretty sure I make chicken cutlets twice a week, especially during the busy ones!

FOR THE ROASTED RED PEPPER MAYO

¾ cup mayonnaise

¼ cup chopped jarred roasted
   red peppers

4 fresh basil leaves

½ teaspoon kosher salt

⅛ teaspoon crushed red pepper flakes

FOR THE CUTLETS

1½ cups Italian-style bread crumbs

3 tablespoons finely grated Parmigiano-
   Reggiano cheese

1 teaspoon garlic powder

½ teaspoon kosher salt

¼ teaspoon ground black pepper

2 large eggs

4 (4-ounce) thinly sliced boneless, skinless chicken breast cutlets, patted dry

½ cup extra-virgin olive oil

2 cups baby arugula

1 long loaf Italian bread

NOTE

You can add cheese to the sandwiches; mozzarella, Parmesan, and provolone are among the choices.

For Siena, I keep the chicken cutlets plain, though sometimes I will cut the chicken in strips and serve with honey mustard sauce. For Brian and me, I wrap up the sandwiches in parchment paper for us to grab when we need to!

1. **MAKE THE ROASTED RED PEPPER MAYO:** In a food processor fitted with the S blade, process the mayonnaise, red peppers, basil, salt, and red pepper flakes until smooth, scraping down the sides of the bowl as needed. Transfer to a bowl and set aside.

2. **MAKE THE CUTLETS:** In a large shallow bowl, stir together the bread crumbs, Parmigiano cheese, garlic powder, salt, and black pepper. In another shallow bowl, lightly whisk the eggs.

3. Working with one cutlet at a time, dip the chicken in the eggs, coating both sides and letting the excess drip off. Dip in the crumb mixture, turning to fully coat both sides.

4. In a large frying pan over medium heat, warm the oil. When it is hot, add the cutlets, in batches as necessary. Cook, turning once, until the meat is cooked through and the cutlets are golden brown on both sides, about 4 minutes per side. Transfer to a paper towel–lined plate to drain.

5. To assemble the sandwiches, cut the bread into four 4- to 5-inch-long sections, split horizontally in half.

6. Spread about 2 tablespoons of the roasted red pepper mayo on the bottom halves of the bread. Top with a chicken cutlet, a handful of arugula, and the top side of the bread. Serve immediately or wrap tightly and refrigerate overnight.

MORE TO SHARE RECIPE

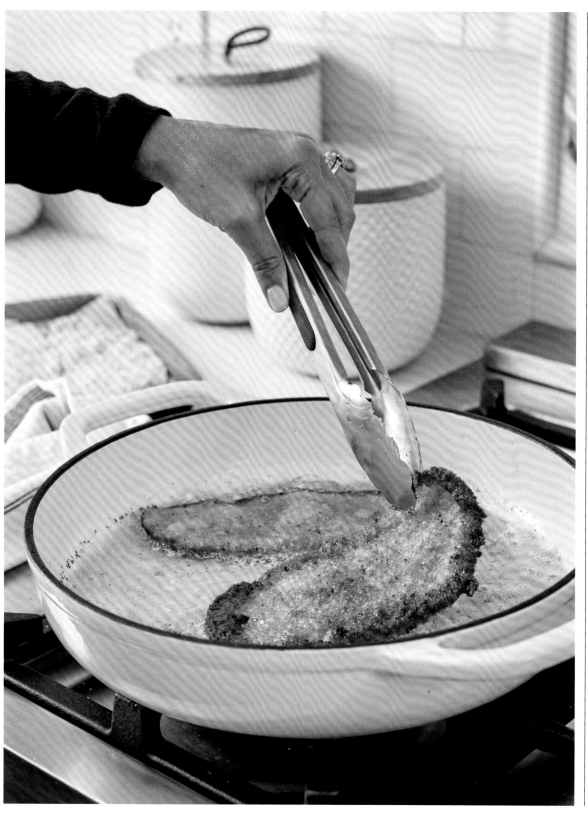

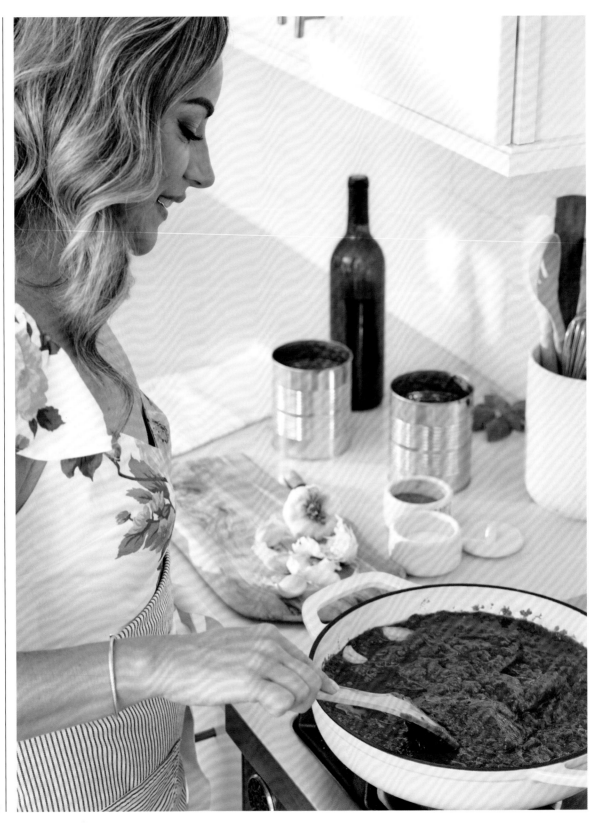

Easy Marinara Sauce

MAKES: ABOUT 3 CUPS | PREP: 5 MINUTES | COOK: 20 MINUTES

It may sound pretentious, but I typically don't use jarred premade tomato sauce. Home-made sauce was something I took for granted growing up. Watching my mom open a can of crushed tomatoes and fry the garlic in oil seemed just as quick and easy to me as opening a jar, and I've kept the habit ever since. If you try making this fresh tomato sauce, I hope the smell of garlic and oil becomes as comforting to you as it is to me.

2 tablespoons extra-virgin olive oil

4 cloves garlic, crushed

1 (28-ounce) can crushed tomatoes, pureed (I use Pastene brand)

¼ cup red wine (optional)

1 tablespoon dried basil

2 teaspoons kosher salt

1 teaspoon ground black pepper

1 teaspoon garlic powder

1. In a medium pan over medium heat, warm the oil. Add the garlic and sauté until golden brown, about 3 minutes.

2. Briefly remove the pan from the heat and carefully add the tomatoes; they may splatter when they hit the hot oil. Return to the stove and stir in the wine (if using). Heat to a simmer, then add the basil, salt, pepper, and garlic powder.

3. Cover the pan and reduce the heat to low. Cook until the sauce thickens, about 15 minutes.

4. Serve the sauce over any type of pasta along with crusty bread for sopping up the extra!

NOTE

Refrigerate the sauce in an airtight container for up to 4 days or freeze for up to 2 months.

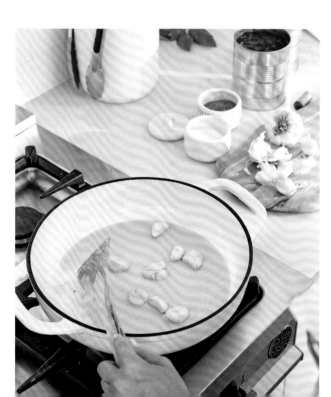

Raise your hand if you feel like you spend 85 percent of your life in the car! It's true, so many of us are commuting or shuttling kids to activities practically around the clock. This is what may have influenced some people to participate in the "car confessions" trend on social media. People sit in their cars, video cameras running, spilling their thoughts on life or current events. Instead of listening to music or a podcast when stuck in traffic or the school drop-off line, people use the time to unload their thoughts.

It makes me think about the time I spend with God. Often when I'm praying, I list out what I need from him and my concerns or hopes for others. I make sure to thank him and offer praise. But what about confession? What about coming face-to-face with our own shortcomings? Sounds like a sure way to get in trouble.

> When I kept silent,
>   my bones wasted away
>   through my groaning all day long.
> For day and night
>   your hand was heavy on me;
> my strength was sapped
>   as in the heat of summer.
>
> PSALM 32:3–4

Sometimes the restlessness we feel can be a signal that we have unfinished business within our hearts or minds. Maybe it's feeling guilty because I shouldn't have ignored my mom's call, but thinking that she knows I am too busy. Or maybe it's feeling bitter that I wasn't chosen for the project I wanted at work, so I decide to slack off. Or I didn't get the lead in the school play, so now I will spend my time gossiping about the person who did. Over time, these feelings pile up, causing extra stress that eventually will catch up with us.

> Then I acknowledged my sin to you
>   and did not cover up my iniquity.

I said, "I will confess
    my transgressions to the LORD."
And you forgave
    the guilt of my sin.

PSALM 32:5

What if, instead of driving our anxious hearts from one place to the next, we stopped and made time for a "car confession"? What if we put ourselves in park and laid it all out on the dashboard?

Talking or venting to a trusted friend can ease our burden, but we can also do the same with God. He is not looking to condemn us but rather to show mercy. To give us confidence to go to a person and rectify a situation. To heal a heart that has been broken by harsh words. To give us words to speak in hard situations. We are not meant to carry all our burdens on our own. There is freedom to be found in honesty before the Lord.

Therefore let all the faithful pray to you
    while you may be found;
surely the rising of the mighty waters
    will not reach them.
You are my hiding place;
    you will protect me from trouble
    and surround me with songs of deliverance.

PSALM 32:6–7

Dear Lord, help me come to you when my heart is heavy. Bring to light that which needs to be forgiven. Let me know confession doesn't lead to condemnation but rather healing. Remove my selfish pride and hardened heart. Give me the wisdom I need to resolve my sin, and let me know I have been forgiven by your unending mercy and grace.

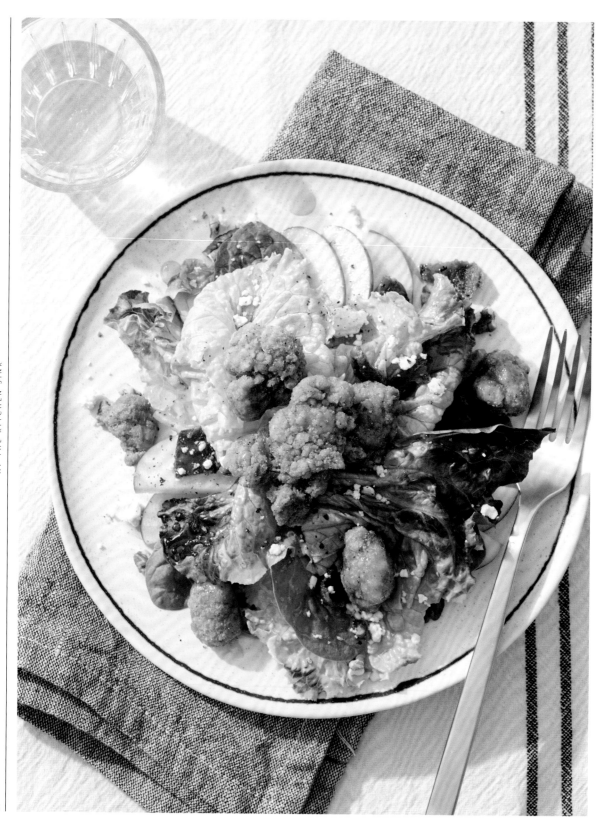

Popcorn Chicken Salad

SERVES: 4 | PREP: 20 MINUTES | COOK: 10 MINUTES | INACTIVE: 10 MINUTES

I am pretty sure most of us have popcorn chicken, or some version of chicken nuggets, stashed in our freezers. When Siena started swimming lessons, we would stop to get takeout at her favorite place once a week. However, I was not as excited to get the crispy nuggets every week, because I was forfeiting the fries for a side salad. I had to do something different. I would still get the nuggets, but I was able to make a large salad with a copycat dressing for Brian and me. This made the trip more budget and adult friendly!

FOR THE VINAIGRETTE

¼ cup extra-virgin olive oil

¼ cup apple cider vinegar

1 tablespoon maple syrup

1 tablespoon freshly squeezed orange juice

1 teaspoon minced shallot

½ teaspoon kosher salt

¼ teaspoon chopped fresh tarragon

⅛ teaspoon ground black pepper

FOR THE SALAD

4 slices thick-cut bacon

6 cups chopped mixed salad greens (such as baby spinach, romaine, and red leaf lettuce)

1 cup chopped green cabbage

2 Honeycrisp apples, chopped

½ cup pecans, chopped

2 ounces crumbled goat cheese

1 (12-ounce) package popcorn chicken, cooked according to package directions

1. **MAKE THE VINAIGRETTE:** In a small bowl, whisk together the oil, vinegar, maple syrup, orange juice, shallot, salt, tarragon, and pepper. Set aside.

2. **MAKE THE SALAD:** Heat a large skillet over medium heat. Add the bacon and cook until crispy, 4 to 5 minutes per side. Transfer to a cutting board. When it is cool enough to handle, chop it into crumbles and set aside.

3. In a large serving bowl, toss the greens, cabbage, apples, pecans, and 3 tablespoons of the vinaigrette until well coated. Add the goat cheese, bacon crumbles, and an additional tablespoon of the vinaigrette and toss gently to evenly mix and coat the ingredients. Top with the popcorn chicken and serve immediately.

Shrimp Scampi over Linguine

SERVES: 6 | PREP: 15 MINUTES | COOK: 20 MINUTES | INACTIVE: 15 MINUTES

Although shrimp scampi sounds like a fancy restaurant dish, it was a go-to meal when Brian and I were newly married. I was coming home from interning or working at the school, and sometimes had only an hour before I had to head out again to grad school classes. This dish always felt like a complete meal and is ready to serve in about 20 minutes. Pair this with a glass of wine on a Friday night, and it's a date!

FOR THE SHRIMP

1 pound large (26- to 30-count) raw shrimp, peeled and deveined

2 tablespoons extra-virgin olive oil

½ teaspoon finely chopped garlic

½ teaspoon kosher salt

Ground black pepper

FOR THE PASTA

Kosher salt

1 (1-pound) box linguine

4 tablespoons unsalted butter

¼ cup extra-virgin olive oil, plus more for serving

¼ cup finely chopped shallots

2 tablespoons finely chopped garlic

¼ teaspoon crushed red pepper flakes, plus more for serving (optional)

½ cup dry white wine

Juice of 1 lemon

Ground black pepper

¼ cup loosely packed fresh parsley, chopped

1. **PREPARE THE SHRIMP:** In a medium bowl, toss the shrimp with the oil, garlic, salt, and pepper to evenly coat the shrimp. Let marinate for 15 minutes.

2. **MAKE THE PASTA:** Bring a large pot of water to a boil, then add 1 tablespoon of the salt and the linguini. Cook until the pasta is al dente, 8 to 9 minutes. Drain well, reserving ¼ cup of the cooking water.

3. Meanwhile, in a large high-sided sauté pan over medium heat, melt 2 tablespoons of the butter with 2 tablespoons of the oil. Add the shallots, garlic, and red pepper flakes (if using) and sauté until the shallots are translucent, about 3 minutes.

4. Increase the heat to medium-high and add the shrimp. Cook, turning them once or twice, until the shrimp turn pink, about 3 minutes. Remove from the pan and set aside.

5. With the pan over medium heat, add the wine, lemon juice, and reserved pasta water and bring to a boil. Add the remaining 2 tablespoons each of butter and oil, cooking just until the butter melts. Season with salt and pepper to taste.

6. Add the shrimp, pasta, and parsley to the sauce, stirring to coat.

7. Serve immediately with a drizzle of oil and a pinch of red pepper flakes (if using).

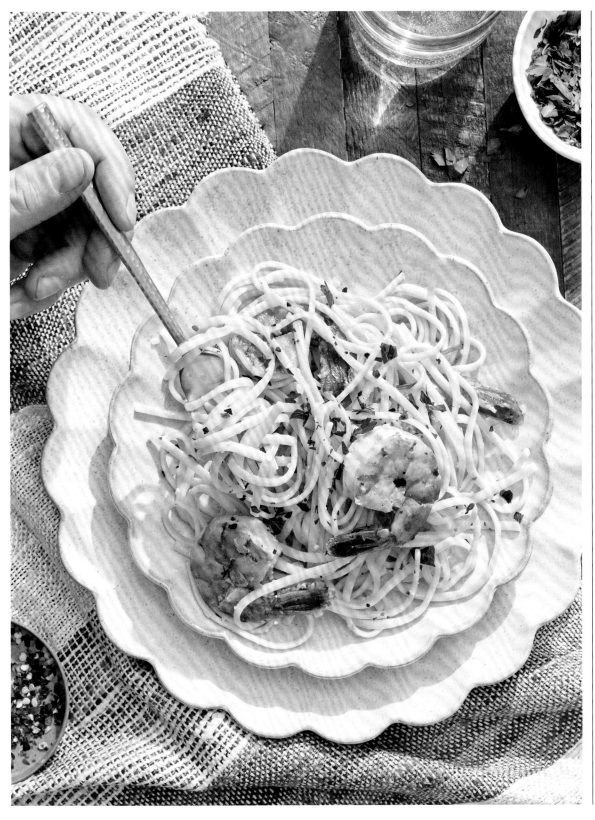

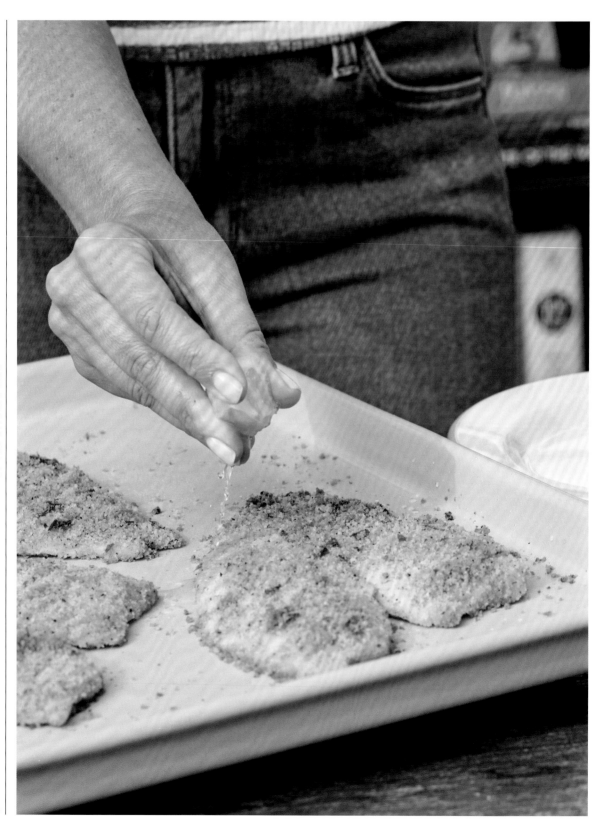

Baked Lemon Garlic~Crusted Flounder

SERVES: 4 | PREP: 10 MINUTES | COOK: 15 MINUTES | INACTIVE: 5 MINUTES

Telling people my daughter eats baked flounder never gets old. In truth, it's an elevated version of a fish stick, so maybe I shouldn't be overly proud. However, it is possible this dish will convert your family into fish lovers. Using a Microplane to zest garlic and lemon into the bread crumbs is the secret weapon here. Also, the fact that this comes together in 30 minutes makes it a weeknight winner!

4 (8-ounce) flounder fillets

¾ cup Italian-style bread crumbs

¼ cup freshly grated Parmigiano-Reggiano cheese

1½ teaspoons finely chopped fresh basil

½ teaspoon kosher salt, plus more as needed

⅛ teaspoon ground black pepper

1½ teaspoons minced garlic

1 teaspoon lemon zest

3 tablespoons extra-virgin olive oil, plus more for baking

Lemon wedges, for serving

1. Preheat the oven to 400°F. Line a baking sheet with parchment paper.

2. In a large shallow bowl, stir together the bread crumbs, cheese, basil, ½ teaspoon salt, and the pepper. Add the garlic and lemon zest and mix to combine.

3. Add the oil, 1 tablespoon at a time, mixing well between each addition. When all the oil has been added, the mixture should be the consistency of wet sand.

4. Dredge each flounder fillet in the bread crumb mixture, coating both sides and gently pressing the crumbs in place. Arrange the fillets on the prepared baking sheet and spoon any remaining crumbs over the top. Drizzle lightly with oil.

5. Bake the fish until it is cooked through and the crumbs are golden brown, about 15 minutes. Let rest for 5 minutes.

6. Serve with lemon wedges and a sprinkle of kosher salt.

Roasted Broccoli with Honey

Siena thinks something is wrong with broccoli when it is served steamed or raw. I am not sure if that is good or bad, but I consider it a win that she eats up this roasted broccoli a couple of times a week! Sometimes I will change things up and serve this broccoli with a Caesar dressing. Or I'll give it a rough chop and add it to pasta.

2 heads broccoli, cut into florets

3 tablespoons extra-virgin olive oil

1 teaspoon kosher salt, plus more for serving

¼ teaspoon ground black pepper

2 teaspoons honey

1. Preheat the oven to 425°F. Line a large baking sheet with parchment paper.

2. Spread the broccoli florets on the prepared baking sheet. Drizzle with the oil and add the salt and pepper. Toss to coat the broccoli with oil, then spread the florets evenly over the baking sheet.

3. Roast the broccoli about 10 minutes. Turn the florets and continue roasting until they turn deep brown in color, about 10 minutes more.

4. To serve, drizzle the honey evenly over hot broccoli and sprinkle lightly with salt.

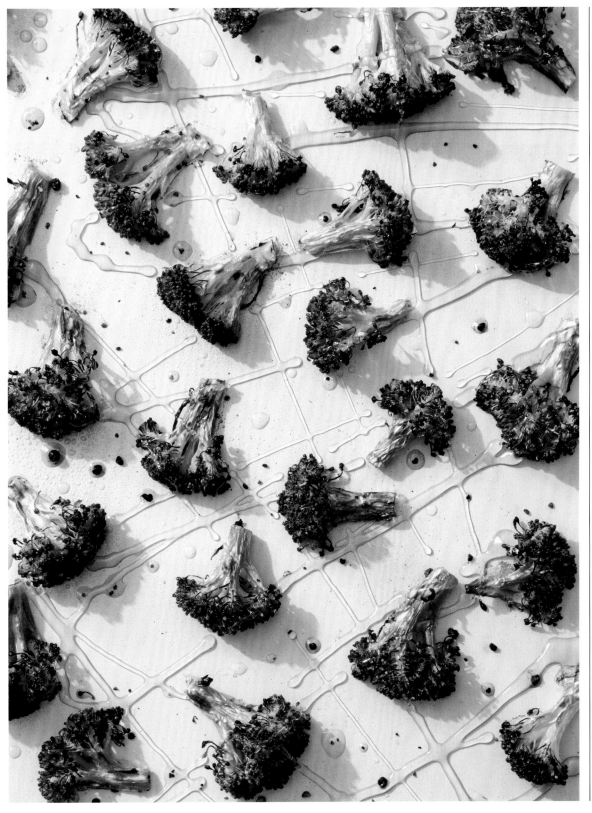

6

Pantry Picks: Something from Nothing

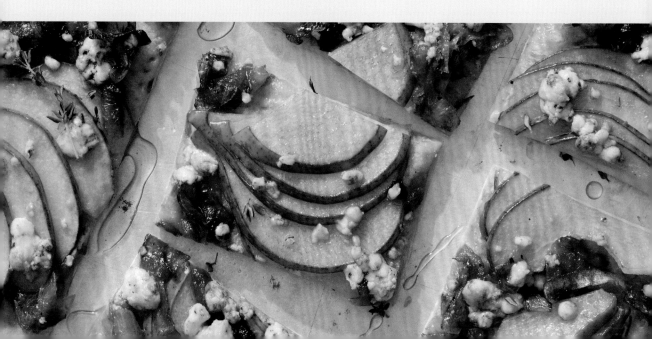

One Sunday, our extended family didn't have plans for our regular get-together. Schedules were last-minute, and no one could decide where to go.

When I host, I normally like to have a solid plan. To build it, I think through the menu and make an extra shopping trip during the week. However, as I looked around my kitchen that day, I started to see that I had what I needed to pull off Sunday dinner. In the fridge, I spotted a package of chicken breasts that could be turned into crispy cutlets for the kids. On the counter, I spied cherry tomatoes that could become fresh tomato sauce. And a wheel of Brie I hadn't used for recipe testing would pair perfectly with the grapes Siena hadn't eaten and crackers I always keep in the pantry. Instant cheese board! With that, I felt confident I could pull off dinner. I told everyone to come on over, and then I got to work.

Too often, we forget that God made us in his image, that he loves us and created us with purpose. Instead, we buy into the mythology that we have nothing of significance to offer. Let yourself be encouraged as you realize God can make something out of what you perceive to be nothing. If he can use the widow's last mite and feed five thousand people with a little boy's lunch, what can he do through you?

Jesus replied, "They do not need to go away. You give them something to eat."

"We have here only five loaves of bread and two fish," they answered.

"Bring them here to me," he said. And he directed the people to sit down on the grass. Taking the five loaves and the two fish and looking up to heaven, he gave thanks and broke the loaves. Then he gave them to the disciples, and the disciples gave them to the people. They all ate and were satisfied, and the disciples picked up twelve basketfuls of broken pieces that were left over.

MATTHEW 14:16–20

Too often we think we need to have everything in perfect order to be successful. We need to have our tables and homes in perfect shape, and we fear that guests will notice the dust on the top shelf or that the serving platters do not match. We think that maybe they'll gossip about our furniture that clearly doesn't belong in a Pottery Barn catalog or that they'll secretly loathe our version of chicken Parmesan. This attitude causes us to miss the simplicity of the situation. The part where, if we are obedient to what God has asked us to do, he will take care of the rest.

What if Jesus bought into the disciples' perception of scarcity regarding the five loaves and two fishes? What if he said, "You're right, a couple of loaves of bread aren't going to feed a hangry crowd"? As an Italian American whose greatest fear is running out of food at a gathering, I understand.

The disciples saw the problem, but Jesus saw what was possible. The child's small act of obedience—sharing his food—yielded worthwhile results. Sometimes God asks us to take what we have and use it, regardless of how it looks or feels to us. He can take what we write off as nothing and turn it into something meaningful.

Last-minute dinners fill my heart and home with joy. They aren't perfectly planned and my menu isn't always well thought out, but those gatherings always serve a purpose. Sometimes when we get out of our own way and let God have his, we open ourselves up to unexpected joy. I'll hear the kids laughing in the basement, and it soothes my soul. I'll clean up with my mom and sisters, and revel in the heart-filling conversations. All because I've chosen to look at what I had to offer instead of focusing on what I didn't have. I'm sensing I should do more of this, focusing on what I must give and letting God take care of the rest.

———————

Dear Lord, please help me keep my heart open to the blessings that are right in front of me. Help me recognize that perfection is not a prerequisite to joy. Help me to be flexible and adaptable where I need to be instead of rigid and anxious. Soften my heart and open my eyes to the abundance that surrounds me through you.

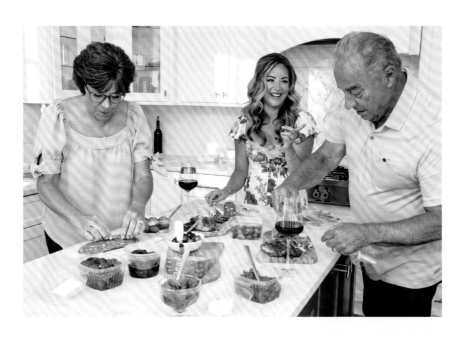

Pasta Puttanesca

SERVES: 4 | PREP: 10 MINUTES | COOK: 25 MINUTES

If you do not know the origins of pasta puttanesca, then let me fill you in. They say this dish may have been invented in Naples by the "women of the night." (When I included this fun fact in one of my first church conference speaking engagements, I received a lot of laughs and a couple of raised eyebrows.) Whatever the recipe's origins, this quick pasta dish is one of my personal favorites. It is one of the reasons why I always keep a jar of olives in the pantry. Don't be afraid to use the olive brine as an ingredient in the sauce! Better yet, save the brine to marinate chicken or fish!

1 tablespoon kosher salt plus one teaspoon

1 (1-pound) box spaghetti or bucatini

2 tablespoons extra-virgin olive oil

3 garlic cloves, finely chopped

4 to 5 anchovy fillets in oil plus 1 teaspoon oil from the tin

2 tablespoons capers, drained

1 (28-ounce) can crushed tomatoes, pureed

1¼ cups pitted Kalamata olives

1 teaspoon crushed red pepper flakes

1 teaspoon dried oregano

½ teaspoon ground black pepper

Crusty bread, for serving (optional)

Slivered fresh basil, for serving (optional)

1. Bring a large pot of water to a boil. Add 1 tablespoon salt and the spaghetti. Cook until al dente, 8 to 9 minutes. Drain well, reserving ½ cup of the pasta water.

2. Meanwhile, in a large sauté pan over medium heat, warm the olive oil. Add the garlic and anchovies and sauté until the garlic cloves start to turn golden brown, about 3 minutes.

3. Turn the heat to medium-low and add the anchovy oil and capers; sauté for 1 minute. Stir in the tomatoes, olives, red pepper flakes, oregano, the remaining 1 teaspoon of salt, and pepper.

4. Bring to a gentle simmer. Cover and cook for 15 minutes, allowing the flavors to develop. Season with additional salt and pepper to taste.

5. Add the pasta and reserved cooking water to the pan, tossing to coat the pasta with sauce.

6. Serve with bread and fresh basil (if using).

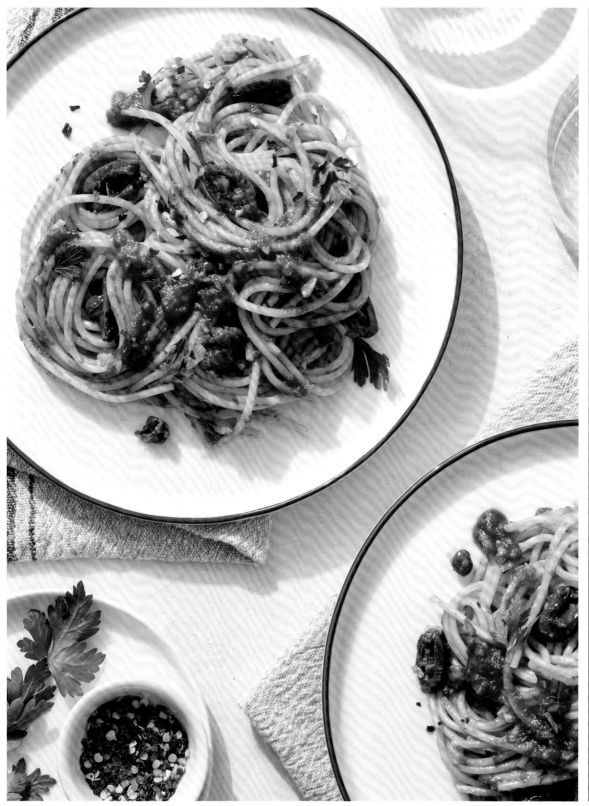

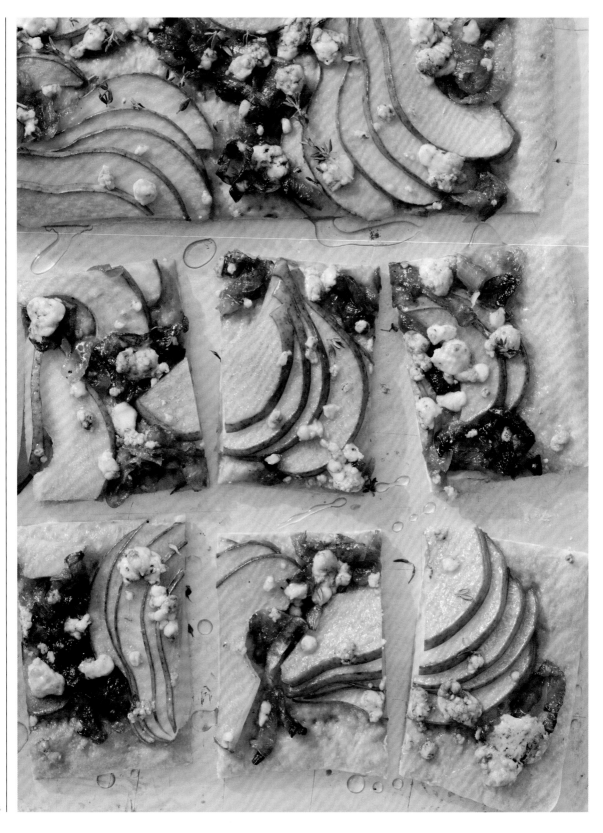

Pear and Gorgonzola Flatbread

SERVES: 4 TO 6 | PREP: 15 MINUTES | COOK: 45 MINUTES

This recipe is on repeat during the holiday season when I need something to bring to gatherings. Using the ready-made pizza crust helps it come together quicker. The crust has a bit of sweetness to it that traditional pizza crusts do not. However, this unexpected flavor is what makes the flatbread so good. Also, the can of pizza crust is easy to keep in the fridge and have on hand for surprise guests.

3 tablespoons unsalted butter

1 yellow onion, thinly sliced into half moons

1½ teaspoons kosher salt

½ teaspoon sugar

1 (13- to 14-ounce) can refrigerated pizza crust (I like Pillsbury Classic)

2 tablespoons extra-virgin olive oil

1 tablespoon balsamic vinegar

1½ teaspoons honey

⅛ teaspoon ground black pepper

2 ripe Bartlett pears, cored and thinly sliced

½ cup crumbled gorgonzola cheese

1. In a large high-sided skillet over medium heat, melt the butter. Add the onions and toss to coat with the butter. Sauté, stirring frequently, about 15 minutes. Add 1 teaspoon of the salt and the sugar and stir to combine. Lower the heat to medium-low and sauté, stirring occasionally, until the onions turn a rich, golden color, 10 to 15 minutes more. Remove from the heat.

2. Preheat the oven to 400°F.

3. On a large baking sheet, roll out the pizza crust, using your fingers to gently spread the dough toward the edges of the pan. Use a fork to prick the entire surface of the dough.

4. In a small bowl, whisk together the oil, vinegar, honey, the remaining ½ teaspoon of salt, and the pepper. Using a pastry brush, brush some of the mixture over the top of the dough.

5. Leaving a ½-inch border around the edges, arrange the pear slices over the dough, shingling them slightly. Brush with the remaining oil mixture.

6. Bake for 5 minutes. Carefully spread the onions over the pears and top with the gorgonzola. Return to the oven and bake until the edges are golden brown and the cheese has melted, 10 minutes. Let stand for 5 minutes, then cut into squares. Serve warm or at room temperature.

Artichoke and White Bean Soup

SERVES: 4 | PREP: 20 MINUTES | COOK: 20 MINUTES | INACTIVE: 5 MINUTES

When soup season hits, I love having a batch of this dish in the fridge or the freezer. When I was retesting the recipe for the book, I found myself wanting some extra texture, but I didn't want to throw in croutons. The crispy artichokes were a last-minute decision that was perfect, and they're now a permanent part of the dish. It is almost like topping the soup with the best part of a stuffed artichoke!

FOR THE SOUP

1 tablespoon apple cider vinegar

1 teaspoon Dijon mustard

1 teaspoon honey

1 teaspoon lemon zest

1 teaspoon kosher salt, plus more
as needed

½ teaspoon onion powder

½ teaspoon garlic powder

½ teaspoon ground black pepper,
plus more as needed

2 tablespoons unsalted butter

1 tablespoon chopped garlic

½ cup chopped green onions, white
and green parts

2 (15-ounce) cans cannellini beans,
drained and rinsed

1 (14-ounce) can quartered artichoke
hearts, drained

1 tablespoon extra-virgin olive oil

2 cups chicken broth

1 sprig fresh rosemary

FOR THE CRISPY ARTICHOKES

3 tablespoons extra-virgin olive oil

1 (14-ounce) can quartered artichoke
hearts, drained and chopped

1½ teaspoons chopped green onions,
white and green parts

2½ tablespoons Italian-style
bread crumbs

1. **MAKE THE SOUP:** In a small bowl, whisk together the vinegar, mustard, honey, lemon zest, salt, onion powder, garlic powder, and pepper.

2. In a large Dutch oven over medium heat, melt the butter. Add the garlic and sauté until fragrant, about 30 seconds. Add the green onions and cook, stirring constantly, 2 minutes.

3. Stir in the beans, artichokes, oil, and vinegar mixture. Sauté, stirring often, for 3 minutes.

4. Add the chicken broth and bring to a simmer. Add the rosemary, then cover and simmer to let the flavors develop, 10 minutes.

5. Meanwhile, **MAKE THE CRISPY ARTICHOKES:** In a large frying pan over medium-high heat, warm the oil. Add the artichokes and green onions and cook, stirring several times, about 3 minutes.

6. Sprinkle the bread crumbs evenly over the artichokes and gently toss to coat. Cook, stirring occasionally, until the crumbs and artichokes are crisp and golden, 5 to 7 minutes. Transfer to a plate and set aside.

7. Remove the soup from the heat, uncover, and let cool for 5 to 10 minutes. Carefully remove the rosemary and transfer the mixture to a blender; puree until smooth. Return the puree to the pot. If it seems too thick, add up to ½ cup water to reach the desired consistency. Cook over medium-high heat until warmed through and add salt and pepper to taste.

8. To serve, ladle the soup into serving bowls and top with the crispy artichokes.

MORE TO SHARE RECIPE

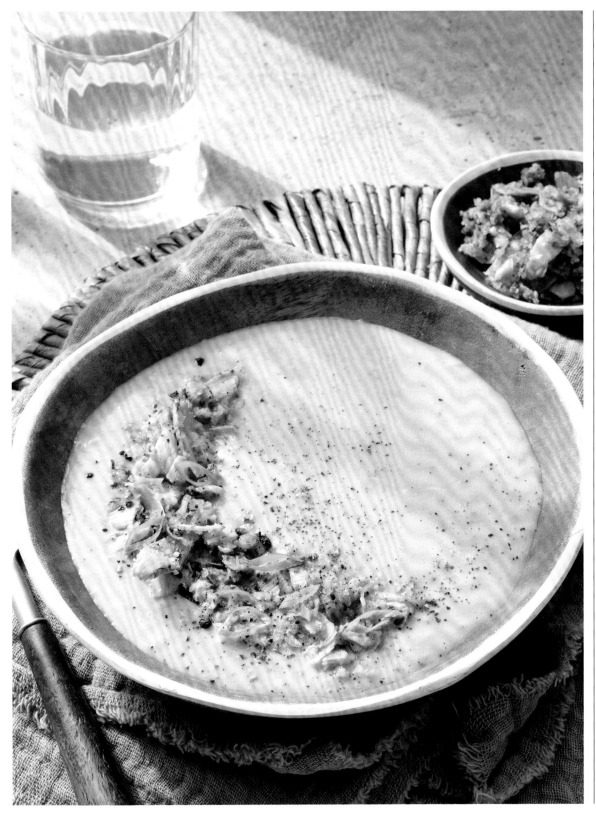

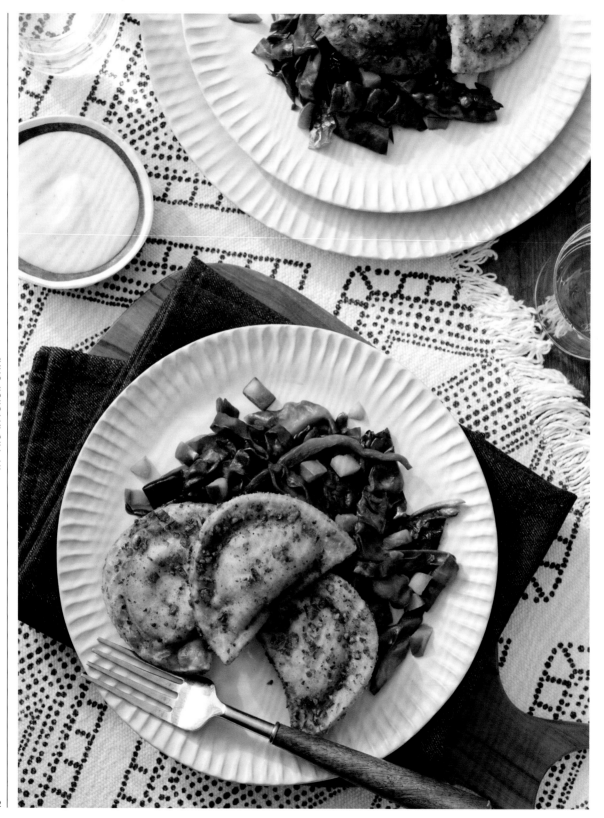

Pretzel-Crusted Pierogies
with Apple Cabbage Sauté

SERVES: 3 TO 4 | PREP: 15 MINUTES | COOK: 20 MINUTES

Don't throw out the crushed-up pretzels at the bottom of the bag! Use them to elevate those pierogies you have stashed in your freezer or fridge. These pretzel-crusted pierogies are also great heated up and put in a Thermos lunch box!

FOR THE HONEY DIJON SAUCE

¼ cup sour cream

3 tablespoons Dijon mustard

1½ tablespoons honey

⅛ teaspoon kosher salt

Pinch of ground black pepper

FOR THE APPLE CABBAGE SAUTÉ

1 tablespoon unsalted butter

½ head of purple cabbage, shredded (about 6 cups)

½ teaspoon kosher salt

⅛ teaspoon ground black pepper

1 medium crisp apple such as Gala, chopped (about 1 cup)

FOR THE PIEROGIES

2 cups salted mini pretzels

½ cup all-purpose flour

1 teaspoon ground mustard

2 large eggs

Extra-virgin olive oil, for cooking

1 (13-ounce) package potato pierogies, thawed

1. **MAKE THE HONEY DIJON SAUCE:** In a small bowl, whisk together the sour cream, mustard, honey, salt, and pepper until well combined. Set aside.

2. **MAKE THE APPLE CABBAGE SAUTÉ:** In a large sauté pan over medium-high heat, melt the butter. Add the cabbage and sauté, stirring often, until it is softened, about 4 minutes. Season with salt and pepper to taste. Mix in the apples and continue to sauté, stirring often, until the apples begin to brown, about 4 minutes more.

3. **MAKE THE PIEROGIES:** In a food processor fitted with the S blade, pulse the pretzels until they're broken into small, uniform-size pieces. Add the flour and ground mustard and pulse until the mixture is fully mixed into coarse crumbs. Transfer the crumbs to a large shallow bowl.

4. Place the eggs in another shallow bowl and whisk.

5. In a large high-sided frying pan over medium-high heat, add oil to a depth of ⅛ inch.

6. Working one at a time, coat the pierogies first in the egg, letting any excess drip off, and then the crumb mixture, turning them over to fully coat both sides. Firmly press them into the crumbs to help them adhere.

7. Carefully add the pierogies to the pan and cook, turning once, until golden brown on each side, about 2 minutes per side. Transfer to a paper towel–lined plate to drain.

8. Divide the pierogis among plates and serve with the apple cabbage sauté and honey Dijon sauce on the side.

NOTE

You can use different types of apples in the sauté recipe. I typically use whatever kind I have on hand.

I usually buy pre-made pierogies in the refrigerator section at the grocery store. They come in a variety of fillings; choose your favorite! If using frozen pierogies, let them thaw and pat them dry before working with them.

When we think of Moses, we typically picture him as a biblical hero, which he absolutely is. We imagine him parting the Red Sea, boldly challenging Pharaoh, saying, "Let my people go!" But Moses is also a reminder that even the greatest heroes among us are prone to the same emotions that affect you and me.

In Exodus 3 and 4, God called on Moses to lead his people out of Egypt, delivering them from Pharaoh and a life of slavery. Moses had his doubts as to why he was assigned this task. In the biblical account, he repeatedly questioned the Lord. Actually, I would say he argued with him:

> Who am I that I should go to
> Pharaoh and bring the Israelites
> out of Egypt?
>
> EXODUS 3:11

Not exactly demonstrating the bold and brave behavior you would think a hero would have, he even tried to convince God to choose somebody else.

Prior to this, God spoke to Moses through a burning bush. I have joked many times that I wish God would just set something on fire in front of me for confirmation. But in Moses's case, it seems, even a miracle wasn't confirmation enough.

Have you ever caught yourself trying to convince God that you are not enough? Or even worse, that he is not enough? We are very good at convincing ourselves that we are not the people for the job. Very quickly, we list our shortcomings. We imagine our failure, convinced we will embarrass ourselves in the end.

> And Moses said to God, Behold, when I come to the
> Israelites and say to them, The God of your fathers has
> sent me to you, and they say to me, What is His name?
> What shall I say to them?
>
> EXODUS 3:13, AMPC

You can almost hear the panic in his voice. Does it sound familiar? *God, I can't speak to that person or that group—I have no formal training. I am not cut out to be a mother—I am always losing my temper. I didn't go to school for that. I am too old or too young for this. I am not strong enough or pretty enough. I do not have the personality for that.*

> And God said to Moses, I AM WHO I AM and WHAT I AM, and I WILL BE WHAT I WILL BE; and He said, You shall say this to the Israelites: I AM has sent me to you!
>
> EXODUS 3:14, AMPC

How powerful is that statement from God? We need to be more concerned about who God is than who we are. You do not have to be enough, because he is. He will present the opportunity, and he will fill in the gaps if you just obey and stretch out your rod.

Sometimes we need to let go of the worry and the rationalizing. We need to stop telling ourselves what we are and aren't capable of. This comes from a fear of failure and a desperate need to control the outcome of every situation. Don't miss a blessing because you are holding on to fear. Instead, tap into who God is and who you are through him: a daughter of the GREAT I AM.

Whenever I start to feel like I am falling short or not enough, when the devil starts to whisper in my ear that I am not dynamic enough or smart enough to speak God's truth, whenever he tells me that I am not qualified to be where God has sent me, I remember this verse. I AM has sent me.

Dear Lord, thank you for your strength when I'm weak. It is not about what I can do but what You can do through me. I pray I would steward whatever you have put before me well, in your name! In moments of fear, doubt, and weakness, help me remember that the GREAT I AM is with me.

Cherry Tomato and Burrata Pasta

SERVES: 6 | PREP: 10 MINUTES | COOK: 20 MINUTES

This pasta is close to my heart. My mom asks me to make it for her pretty much every time I stop over for a weekday visit. When I appeared on *Guy's Grocery Games,* I made this in the second round. It's also my favorite dish to make myself when I have the rare chance to be eating dinner by myself. The burrata added at the end just sends this over the edge that I will happily go over!

Kosher salt

1 (1-pound) box spaghetti

½ cup extra-virgin olive oil, plus more for serving

2½ pints cherry tomatoes

2 tablespoons finely chopped garlic

¼ teaspoon ground black pepper

¼ teaspoon sugar

1 teaspoon lemon zest

½ cup chopped fresh basil

4 (4-ounce) balls burrata cheese

1. Bring a large pot of water to a boil. Add 1 tablespoon of salt and the spaghetti. Cook until the pasta is al dente, 9 to 10 minutes. Drain, reserving 1 cup of the pasta water.

2. Meanwhile, in a large high-sided sauté pan over medium-high heat, warm the oil. Add the tomatoes and sauté for 2 minutes. Stir in the garlic, pepper, sugar, and ½ teaspoon salt. Cook, stirring several times, until the tomatoes start to wrinkle and release their juices, about 8 minutes.

3. Using the back of a wooden spoon, gently press any whole tomatoes to help them burst. Stir in ½ cup of the reserved pasta cooking water and bring to a simmer. Add the lemon zest and simmer for 3 minutes. Add salt to taste.

4. Add the pasta and basil and toss to combine. The pasta should be lightly coated with a silky tomato sauce. If it seems dry, add the remaining pasta cooking water, by the tablespoon, to reach the desired consistency.

5. To serve, divide the pasta evenly into serving bowls, spooning some of the cherry tomato sauce over the top. Cut each ball of burrata in half, place in the center of each serving, and drizzle lightly with oil.

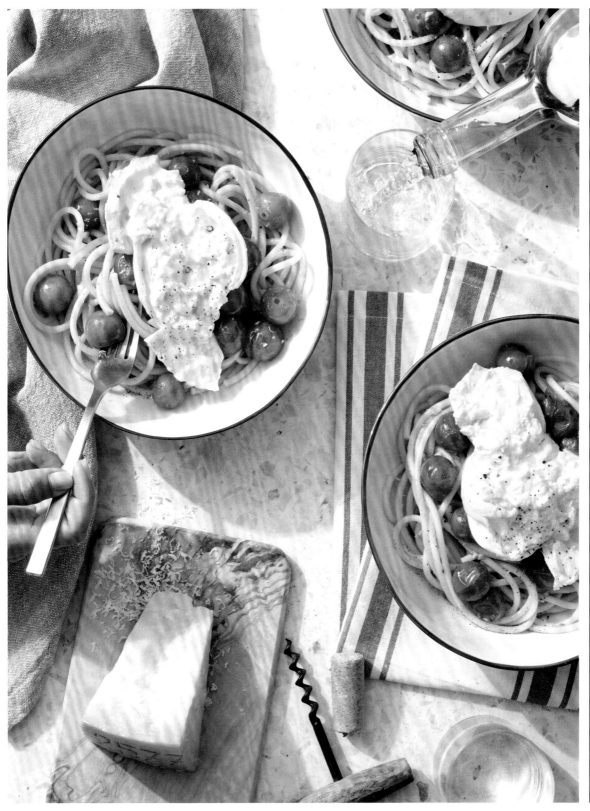

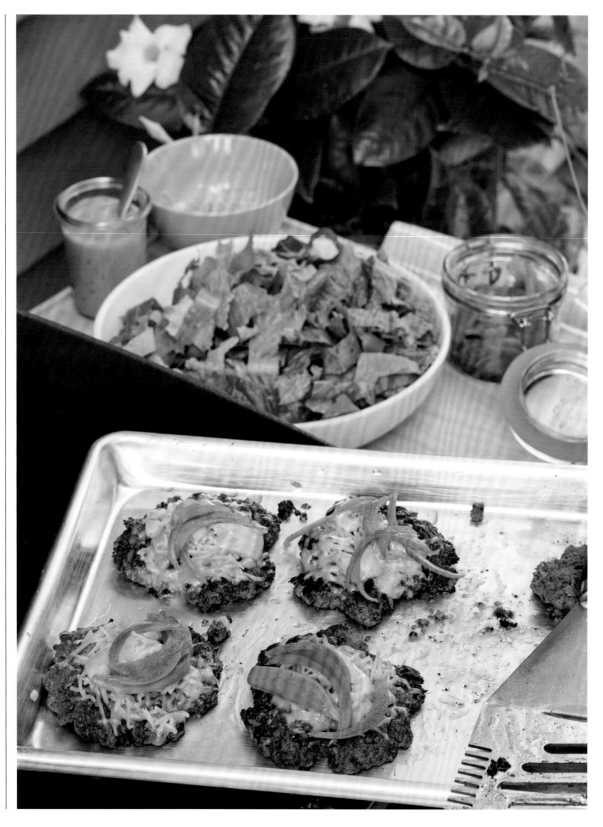

Smash Burger Salad

SERVES: 4 TO 6 | PREP: 15 MINUTES | COOK: 5 MINUTES

One of my favorite meals is a classic burger, fries, and shake. This smash burger salad is like a deconstructed version of that meal. The pickled red onions and the sauce make this an irresistible version of that classic. You'll want to make this any time of the year! It also comes together quite quickly.

FOR THE BURGERS

1 pound lean ground beef (I use 80% lean for the burgers)

2 tablespoons ketchup

1 tablespoon soy sauce

1½ teaspoons Worcestershire sauce

1 teaspoon onion powder

1 teaspoon kosher salt, plus more for sprinkling

½ teaspoon ground black pepper

Unsalted butter, for preparing the griddle

Nonstick cooking spray

FOR THE SAUCE

¾ cup ketchup

½ cup mayonnaise

¼ cup sweet relish

2 tablespoons extra-virgin olive oil

½ teaspoon kosher salt

⅛ teaspoon ground black pepper

FOR THE SALAD

1 head romaine lettuce, chopped

1 cup halved cherry tomatoes

¾ cup shredded Cheddar cheese

½ cup Quick Pickled Red Onions (page 210)

1. **MAKE THE BURGERS:** Working in a large bowl, use your hands to mix the ground beef, ketchup, soy sauce, Worcestershire sauce, onion powder, salt, and pepper until well combined. Divide the meat into five equal portions. Roll each portion into a ball, place on a plate or tray, and cover with plastic wrap while you prep the sauce and salad.

2. **MAKE THE SAUCE:** In a small bowl, stir together the ketchup, mayonnaise, relish, oil, salt, and pepper.

3. **MAKE THE SALAD:** In a large bowl, toss together the lettuce, cherry tomatoes, cheese, and pickled red onions.

4. To cook the burgers, place a griddle over medium-high heat. When it is hot, coat it with a thin film of butter. Lightly coat the back of a metal or silicone spatula with nonstick cooking spray. Working with one at a time, add a ball of meat to the griddle and press down with the back of the spatula, smashing it into a thin, round patty. Repeat with the remaining meat. Season each patty with a sprinkling of salt. Cook until slightly charred, about 3 minutes. Turn the patties and cook on the other side, about 2 minutes. As they're cooked, transfer the burgers to serving plates.

5. Spread about 2 teaspoons of the sauce on each patty. Add the remaining sauce to the salad mixture and toss to combine. Divide the salad among the plates, piling it on top of the burger patties.

NOTE

If you don't have a griddle, a nonstick frying pan works as well. Just cook the burgers in batches.

If you're out of cooking spray, brushing olive oil on the back of the spatula can help keep the meat from sticking.

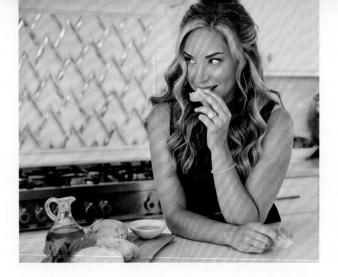

*Now faith is confidence in what we hope for
and assurance about what we do not see.*

HEBREWS 11:1

One sunny day, I took Siena to the playground, as I have many days before. There was a small rock wall that she wanted to climb. It wasn't that high, so I knew she would be able to do it. I had seen her climb taller walls at her gymnastics gym, yet for some reason, she was convinced she could not conquer this one. Every time we went to the playground after that, I would spend at least five minutes reassuring her that she could do it. And then she would decide to skip it, much to my frustration.

One day she started to take a step toward the climb. It seemed she finally decided to trust in her ability and that I would be there if she should fall. That one step turned into a full climb. After that triumph, she now eagerly climbs every structure, even ones I would not like her to!

This situation, as simple as it was, had me thinking of another simple concept. So often, we think we need to come to God with a certain amount of faith. We need to come to him with all our ducks in a row, knowing exactly what we want or need. Or maybe we feel like we need to be more equipped to be in his presence.

*Truly I tell you, if you have faith as small as a
mustard seed, you can say to this mountain,
"Move from here to there," and it will move.
Nothing will be impossible for you.*

MATTHEW 17:20

Have you ever looked at a mustard seed? One of the recipes in this book, Apple Cider Chicken Sandwiches, requires whole-grain mustard. The next time you make it, look at how tiny those seeds are.

As we stare up at the mountain of unbelief, we forget that all we need is a mustard seed of faith to begin. We put so much pressure on ourselves, thinking that we are the be-all and end-all in every situation. This is such a huge mistake! It is the same mistake the disciples made in Matthew 17. A man brought his son to Jesus for healing, explaining that he had previously brought him to the disciples. The disciples were unable to heal him, but Jesus was able to draw the demon out. Later, the disciples came to Jesus asking why they couldn't drive out the demon.

Jesus explained that the disciples were trying to cast out the demon on their own authority and strength, when they should have accessed the power of the Holy Spirit. We need to approach our situations with our faith in Jesus, even if we start with a mustard seed. Have you ever looked up what a mustard seed becomes? It sprouts, then grows into a yellow flowering plant from which pods are harvested. Over time it can spread, growing into a field of yellow blooms, all from a handful of small seeds.

When you are in doubt, ask God to help you find that small seed of faith. You do not have to depend on your own supply. He will multiply and strengthen it. In the midst of your problems, faith and obedience can yield abundance in Jesus's name.

Dear Lord, I thank you that all I need is a small mustard seed of faith. Help my unbelief and my doubt. Nothing is impossible for you. I pray you would move this mountain as only you can.

Tuna and Arugula Salad

SERVES: 4 | PREP: 10 MINUTES

Tuna imported from Italy is different from regular canned tuna. Packed in olive oil, it has a more luxurious feel and richer taste. It can be a bit of a splurge, but it truly is worth it. Flake it into big chunks and turn it into this truly mouthwatering salad that easily one-ups other versions. Brian and I love having it for lunch, and it's also perfect as a light dinner during the summer months out on the deck.

¼ cup extra-virgin olive oil

2 tablespoons red wine vinegar

½ teaspoon Dijon mustard

½ teaspoon kosher salt

⅛ teaspoon ground black pepper

⅛ teaspoon dried oregano

1 (6.7-ounce) jar yellowfin tuna packed in olive oil, preferably from Italy, drained

½ cup chopped, pitted green Cerignola olives

1 cup baby arugula

Shaved Parmigiano-Reggiano cheese, for serving

1. In a medium bowl, whisk together the oil, vinegar, mustard, salt, pepper, and oregano to emulsify.

2. Add the tuna, breaking it into bite-size pieces as you do so. Toss gently to coat it with dressing. Add the olives and arugula and toss until well incorporated.

3. To serve, divide among salad plates and top with shaved Parmigiano cheese.

NOTE

If you do not have shaved Parmigiano cheese, simply leave it off. I would not use grated as it will change the texture of the salad.

The salad can be served on top of a baked flatbread or pizza crust, and finished with an extra drizzle of olive oil. For a delicious sandwich, pile it on crusty bread and spread with a little swipe of Walnut Pesto (214).

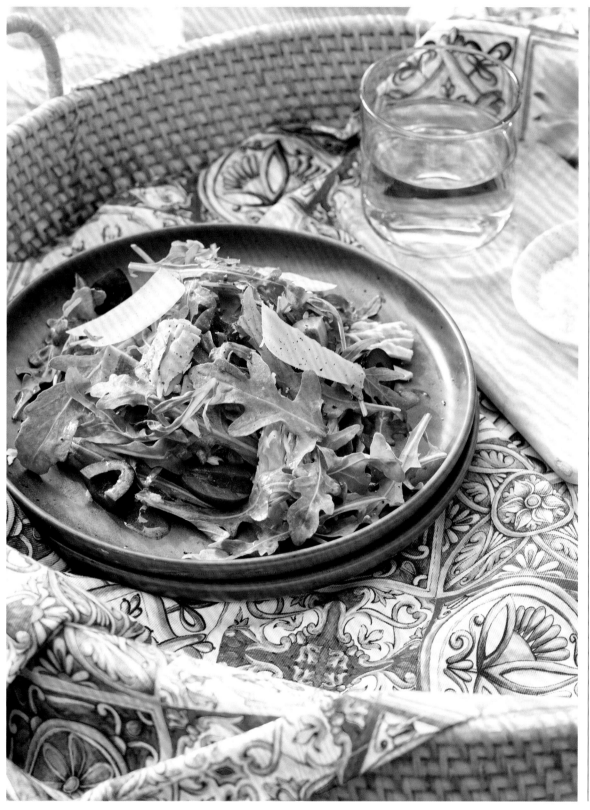

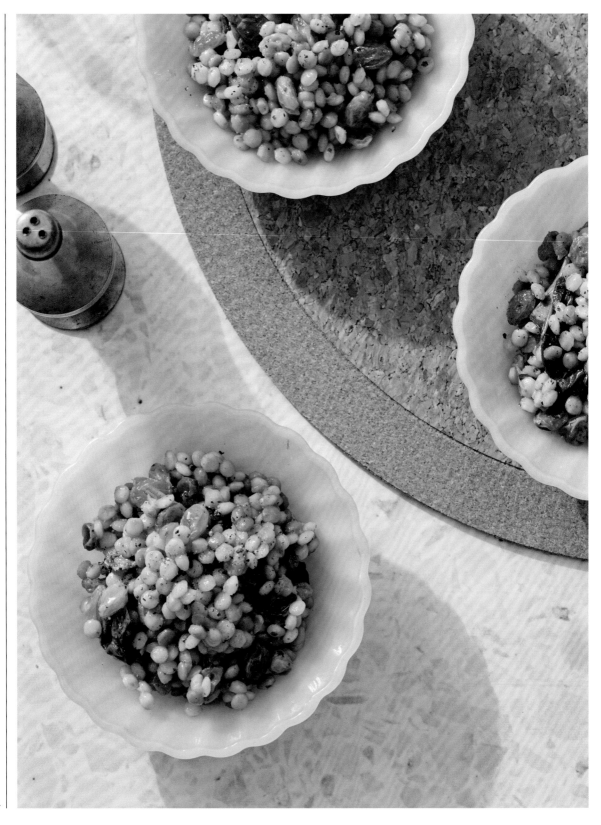

Golden Raisin and Spinach Couscous

MAKES: 2 CUPS | PREP: 10 MINUTES | COOK: 15 MINUTES | INACTIVE: 10 MINUTES

I love couscous or farro. I particularly like using these versatile ingredients as a base for a bowl-type meal. You can toss the grains into salads with arugula, then mix and match the dressings and ingredients to make an interesting side dish any day of the week. This recipe is one of my favorite ways to serve couscous. The golden raisins help encourage kids to try the dish, and the spinach wilted in makes it feel like two dishes in one. On busy weeknights, this is one of my go-to sides.

FOR THE COUSCOUS

1 tablespoon extra-virgin olive oil

¼ cup finely chopped yellow onion

1½ teaspoons kosher salt

1 cup quick-cooking tricolor pearl couscous

1 tablespoon unsalted butter

1 cup fresh baby spinach

½ cup golden raisins

FOR THE DRESSING

¼ cup extra-virgin olive oil

2 tablespoons balsamic vinegar

1 tablespoon honey

1 teaspoon Dijon mustard

1 teaspoon lemon zest

½ teaspoon dried parsley

½ teaspoon kosher salt

¼ teaspoon ground black pepper

1. **MAKE THE COUSCOUS:** In a large high-sided sauté pan over medium-high heat, heat the oil. Add the onions and sauté, stirring several times, until translucent, 5 minutes.

2. Add 1½ cups cold water and the salt and bring to a boil. Stir in the couscous and butter. Reduce to a simmer, cover, and cook until the couscous is tender, about 8 minutes. Remove from the heat and let stand, covered, for 5 minutes.

3. Meanwhile, **MAKE THE DRESSING:** In a large serving bowl, whisk together the oil, vinegar, honey, mustard, lemon zest, parsley, salt, and pepper.

4. Using a fork, fluff the couscous and add it to the dressing in the bowl. Add the spinach and toss together lightly, allowing it to wilt from the heat of the couscous. Add the raisins and mix until the ingredients are well coated with the dressing. Let stand for 5 minutes before serving.

NOTE

Couscous tends to absorb dressing, so taste for seasoning before serving. I usually serve this with a little bit more honey drizzled over the top and a sprinkle of kosher salt for good measure.

I frequently use this as a side dish, saving the leftovers for lunch the next day. Mixing in grilled shrimp or chicken makes it a complete meal.

7

The Sit~Down: Impress Without the Stress

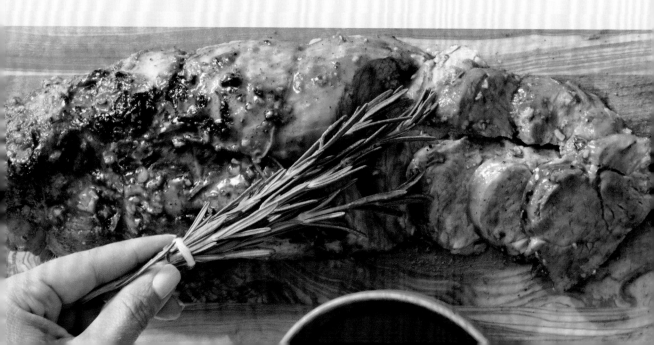

My parents always threw the best parties. Their summer cookouts felt like full-on family reunions. There would be multiple days of kitchen prep and long tables with folding chairs, cordial trays, antipasto platters, and everything in between. I loved watching them prep. My dad would set up the yard with tables, chairs, and coolers full of different drinks, before heading out to pick up catering. And Mom's trips to Costco were events in and of themselves.

They seemed to do it all with effortless ease, although later in life I learned how exhausting it can be to have these gatherings. Inviting others into our home helps build the foundation for family and community. However, the thought of entertaining can be intimidating. We get caught up in the details and perceived shortcomings, worried people will judge our homes and offerings. We compare our tables to the perfectly set ones we see on social media. The organized playrooms with beige-only toys flood our feeds, making us feel like a mess. We worry that someone is going to find dust on a baseboard.

Worrying about these things keeps us isolated and misses the point of gathering. The importance should be on the things that hold real value—time spent together, along with the memories that are being made. This is what helps cultivate a family life, not the perceived perfection pinned on Pinterest feeds.

For I was hungry and you gave me something to eat, I was thirsty and you gave me something to drink, I was a stranger and you invited me in. . . . Truly I tell you, whatever you did for one of the least of these brothers and sisters of mine, you did for me.

MATTHEW 25:35, 40

My mother and I talk on the phone just about every day. During one conversation, she described herself in a way that struck me. We were talking about having people over, whether it be friends or larger family gatherings, and all the work these events take. When I asked if she enjoyed doing it, she said, "Well, I am the one cooking and cleaning up around everyone." She implied that she was not important to the occasion because her efforts were invisible.

It isn't easy to be the host. Having done it myself as an adult, I can understand that now. But it all contributes to fostering lasting relationships, which is at the heart of why we do it. And there's nothing unimportant about that.

Her words sat in the back of my mind. After that conversation, I thought about our family gatherings throughout the years: all the cookouts, the big summer party we would host every August, the countless Sunday dinners my mom has prepared. She had the ability to pull off larger gatherings seamlessly. There was always the perfect amount of food, and then some. There were always enough chairs at the table for whoever wanted to join.

In my eyes, my mom's gift of hospitality was a form of ministry, and there was nothing unimportant about it. However, I'm not sure anyone ever presented it to her that way. Her service hasn't been fueled by competition and isn't for the sake of appearances. It is quite the opposite. She has the willingness to create an environment where people feel comfortable and well taken care of. She takes pride and joy in sharing her home. And yes, she does have a knack for entertaining.

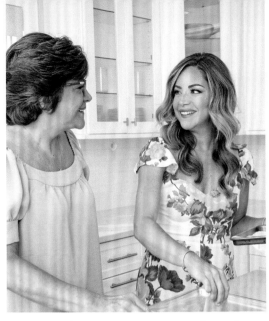

Opening your heart and home takes a lot of work. Sometimes it can feel thankless or inconsequential. However, God sees us and our faithfulness. Not that he wants us to work to the point where we are exhausted and depleted. But he wants us to know that he values our obedience when we use our gifts for him. He doesn't want us to lose sight of our value or worth because we are buying into the world's view of what worth is.

Each of you should use whatever gift you have received to serve others, as faithful stewards of God's grace in its various forms. If anyone speaks, they should do so as one who speaks the very words of God. If anyone serves, they should do so with the strength God provides, so that in all things God may be praised through Jesus Christ. To him be the glory and the power for ever and ever. Amen.

1 PETER 4:10-11

There is so much opportunity to minister in our own homes, families, and communities. It should never be overlooked or undervalued.

Dear Lord, help me see myself as you see me. Shine a light on my God-given talent and give me the motivation and courage to use it for your glory. Let me not lose sight of the fact that you created me with a purpose and that I am worth everything to you.

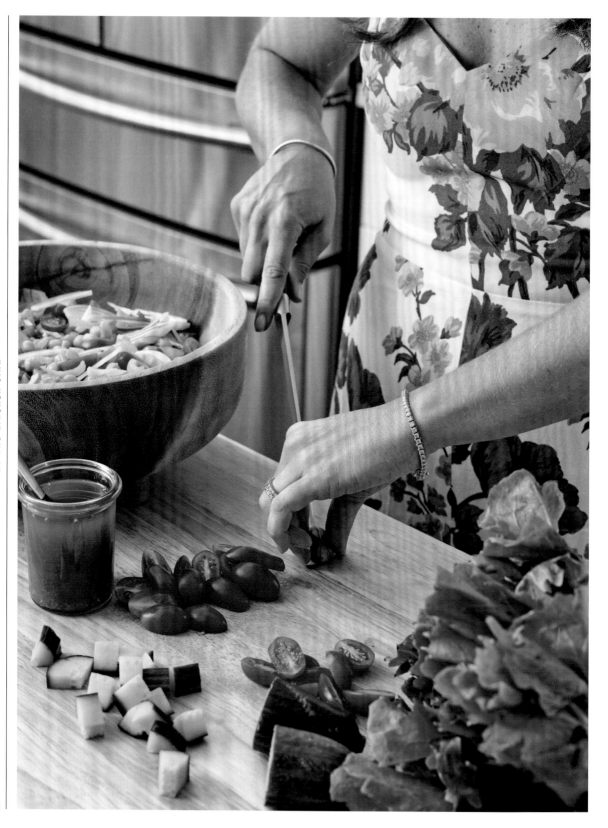

Sunday Dinner Salad

SERVES: 8 | PREP: 15 MINUTES

Our extended family has taken many vacations together. We often find ourselves at the Jersey Shore for long lazy weeks, and we've also enjoyed time in the Bahamas. Each of these places has a Carmine's restaurant nearby and we've made a tradition out of visiting once per trip for an epic family-style dinner. My father orders more than half the menu, and then the biggest plates of pastas and chicken Parmesan fill our table. One of our favorites is the "Carmine" salad chock-full of everything you love about antipasto, plus a great dressing to match. I decided to create a version at home with pantry items. It's now a staple, served almost every Sunday, especially when Baked Penne Vodka (page 178) also is on the menu.

1 cup canned chickpeas, drained

1 cup cherry tomatoes, halved

1 cup chopped cucumbers

½ cup sliced pepperoncini, drained

¼ cup thinly sliced red onion half moons

1 tablespoon extra-virgin olive oil

1 teaspoon red wine vinegar

¼ teaspoon onion powder

¼ teaspoon kosher salt

⅛ teaspoon garlic powder

⅛ teaspoon ground black pepper

1 head escarole, chopped into
   bite-size pieces

½ head red leaf lettuce, chopped into
   bite-size pieces

¼ cup Everyday Dressing (page 213)

1. In a large salad bowl, toss together the chickpeas, tomatoes, cucumbers, pepperoncini, onions, oil, vinegar, onion powder, salt, garlic powder, and pepper.

2. Add the escarole, lettuce, and 2 tablespoons of the dressing and toss gently to combine. Pour the remaining dressing over the top and toss gently to evenly coat the salad with dressing. Serve immediately.

Chicken Marsala
with Pancetta Cream Sauce

SERVES: 4 | PREP: 15 MINUTES | COOK: 50 MINUTES

Both my mom and grandmother love chicken marsala. When I first hosted Mother's Day for them in my first home, I made it for them and they never stopped talking about it. Fast-forwarding a few years, I cooked this family favorite on Hallmark Channel's *Home & Family* after I won its Best Home Cook contest. It's safe to say this dish never disappoints.

FOR THE MUSHROOMS

3 tablespoons unsalted butter

1 garlic clove, chopped

1 heaping tablespoon finely chopped shallots

1 (8- to 10-ounce) container baby bella mushrooms, stems trimmed, sliced ¼ inch thick

Kosher salt

Ground black pepper

FOR THE CHICKEN

1 tablespoon extra-virgin olive oil, plus more as needed

1 (4-ounce) package diced pancetta

1 pound boneless, skinless chicken breast cutlets, patted dry

Kosher salt

Ground black pepper

½ cup all-purpose flour

1 cup sweet Marsala wine

¼ cup heavy cream, plus more, as needed

Chopped flat-leaf parsley, for serving

1. **MAKE THE MUSHROOMS:** In a large skillet over medium heat, melt 2 tablespoons of the butter. Add the garlic and cook, stirring once or twice, until fragrant, 1 minute. Add the shallots and sauté, stirring often until they begin to soften, about 2 minutes.

2. Add the mushrooms and the remaining tablespoon of butter; sauté, shaking the pan occasionally, until softened and lightly browned, about 5 minutes. Add salt and pepper to taste and transfer the mushrooms to a plate.

3. **MAKE THE CHICKEN:** Using the same skillet over medium heat, warm the oil. Add the pancetta and cook, stirring often, until lightly browned and crisp, 6 to 7 minutes. Using a slotted spoon, transfer the pancetta to the plate with the mushrooms, leaving the rendered fat in the pan. Set the pan aside, off the heat.

4. Season both sides of the chicken with salt and pepper. Put the flour in a large shallow bowl. Working with one piece at a time, fully coat both sides of the chicken with flour, shaking off any excess.

5. Return the skillet to medium-high heat. When the oil is hot, fry the chicken in batches, turning once, until it is cooked through and lightly browned on each side, 3 to 4 minutes per side. Transfer the chicken to a plate as it is cooked. Add more oil to the pan as needed and continue frying the chicken.

6. Pour off any excess fat from the skillet and return it to medium-high heat. Add the Marsala, scraping up any browned bits from the bottom of the pan. Bring to a boil and cook until the Marsala reduces by about a quarter of a cup, 2 minutes. Add the cream and cook, stirring often, until it thickens slightly, about 2 minutes.

CONTINUED ON PAGE 154

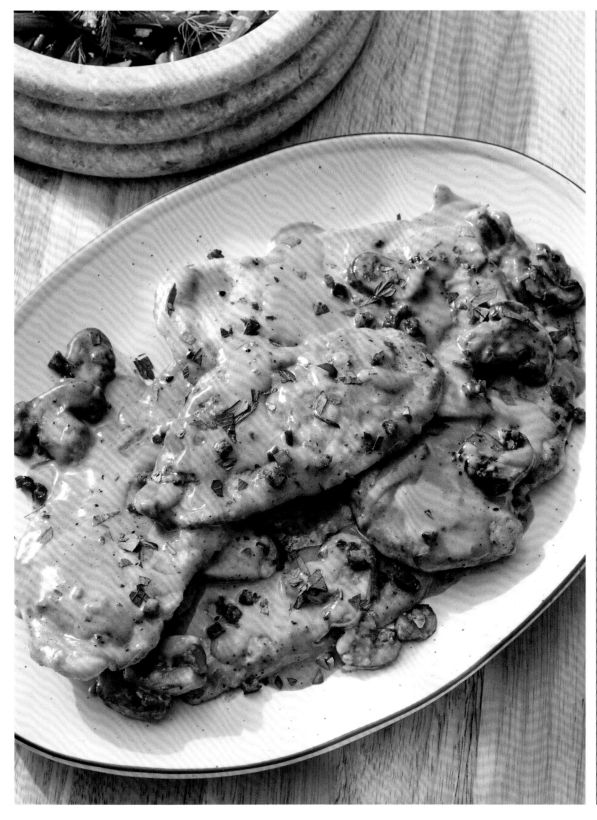

7. Return the chicken, mushrooms, and pancetta to the pan and toss to coat with the sauce. Reduce the heat to low and cook just long enough to warm the chicken and mushrooms. If the sauce is too thick, add more cream by the tablespoon to reach the desired consistency.

8. To serve, spoon the chicken onto plates and top with a portion of mushrooms and sauce. Sprinkle with chopped parsley.

NOTE

Packages of diced pancetta are the easiest option, although you can order a ¼-inch-thick slice from most deli counters and cube it yourself.

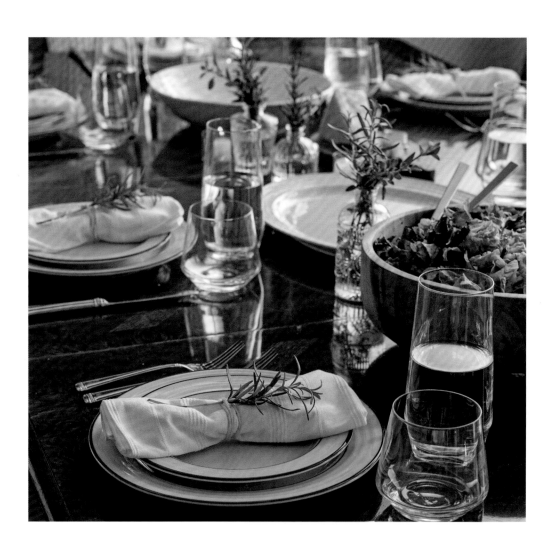

Warm Green Beans
with Feta and Kalamata Olives

SERVES: 4 | PREP: 15 MINUTES | COOK: 10 MINUTES

This quick, classic preparation is taken to the next level with a mixture of fresh, bold, bright flavors. The crispy green beans are complemented by the briny taste of the olives and salty tang of feta cheese. The simple play of textures and flavors creates a stunning vegetable dish that's super easy to make.

Kosher salt

12 ounces trimmed green beans

¾ cup loosely packed fresh dill

½ cup pitted Kalamata olives plus 1½ teaspoons brine from the jar

1 tablespoon lemon zest

1 garlic clove, roughly chopped

½ cup crumbled feta cheese

5 tablespoons extra-virgin olive oil

⅛ teaspoon ground black pepper

1. Bring a large pot of water to a boil. Add 1 teaspoon of salt and the beans. Cook just until they are bright green and crisp-tender, 3 to 4 minutes, depending on their size.

2. While the beans cook, fill a large bowl with ice cubes and water. When the beans are cooked, drain and immediately add them to the ice water to halt the cooking. Drain them and pat dry.

3. In a food processor fitted with the S blade, pulse the dill, olives, lemon zest, and garlic to a coarse, chunky texture, about 10 pulses. Transfer the mixture to a large serving bowl and add the feta, 3 tablespoons of the oil, and the olive brine.

4. In a large sauté pan over medium-high heat, warm the remaining 2 tablespoons of oil. Add the beans, 1 teaspoon of salt, and the pepper. Cook, stirring several times, until they're heated through, 2 to 3 minutes.

5. Add the beans to the serving bowl and toss gently to combine. Serve warm.

Smashed Potatoes
with Crispy Capers

SERVES: 4 TO 6 | PREP: 15 MINUTES | COOK: 1 HOUR 5 MINUTES | INACTIVE: 15 MINUTES

I find I make these potatoes even more often than a baked potato. They are crispy and salty, and I never have any left over when I serve them at larger gatherings. The potatoes are boiled in white vinegar and paired with briny capers. The combination may remind you of salt and vinegar potato chips, only not quite as potent.

1 pound baby yellow potatoes

1 cup distilled white vinegar

1 tablespoon plus ¼ teaspoon kosher salt, plus more for serving

¼ cup extra-virgin olive oil

2 tablespoons capers, drained

1 teaspoon Dijon mustard

½ teaspoon honey

¼ teaspoon ground black pepper

1. Place the potatoes in a large pot. Add the vinegar, 1 tablespoon of the salt, and cold water to cover. Over high heat, bring to a boil and cook until the potatoes are fork-tender, 18 to 20 minutes, depending on size. Drain and set aside.

2. Preheat the oven to 425°F.

3. In a small bowl, whisk together the oil, capers, mustard, honey, the remaining ¼ teaspoon of salt, and the pepper.

4. Arrange the potatoes on a large rimmed baking sheet. Using a potato masher or the bottom of a heavy glass, press down on each potato until they're smashed into broken-edged rounds about ½ inch thick.

5. Brush each potato with the olive oil mixture. You will not use all of it; reserve the unused oil.

6. Bake for 15 minutes. Remove the pan from the oven and spoon the remaining olive oil mixture over the top of each potato, leaving the capers behind. Give the pan a gentle shake to help distribute, then return them to the oven and bake for 15 minutes more.

7. Spoon the capers over and around the potatoes and bake until the potatoes are golden brown and crispy around the edges, about 10 minutes more. Sprinkle with salt and serve.

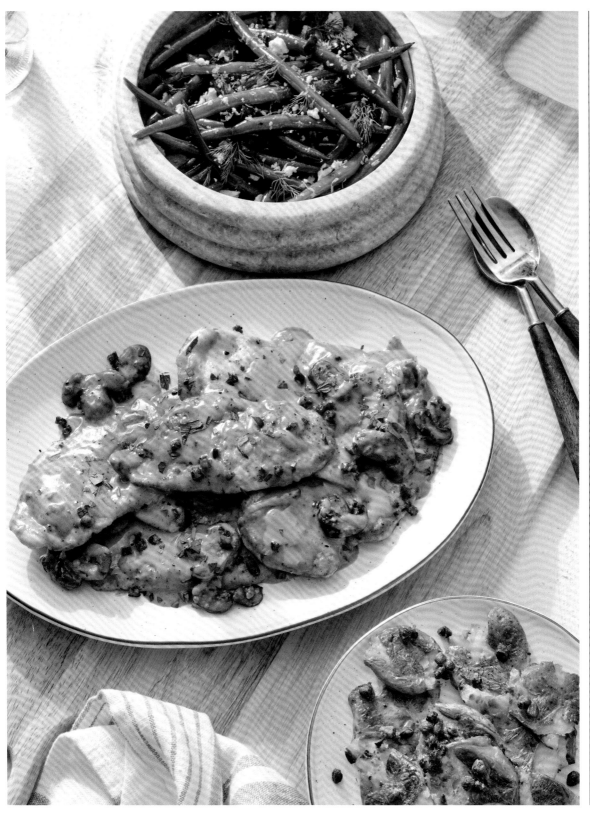

Sautéed Brussels Sprouts
with Pancetta

SERVES: 4 | PREP: 5 MINUTES | COOK: 15 MINUTES

This crispy brussels sprouts dish has become one of my favorites for holidays and Sunday dinners. It seems to make kids and adults equally happy. The flavor is salty and sweet—definitely not the old-school brussels sprouts that people dread.

2 tablespoons extra-virgin olive oil

1 (4-ounce) package diced pancetta

1 (12-ounce) bag shaved
 brussels sprouts

2 tablespoons freshly squeezed
 lemon juice

1½ tablespoons apple cider vinegar

½ teaspoon maple syrup

½ teaspoon kosher salt

⅛ teaspoon ground black pepper

1. In a large sauté pan over medium-high heat, warm 1 tablespoon of the oil. Add the pancetta and cook, stirring several times, until crispy and browned, 5 to 7 minutes. Using a slotted spoon, transfer the pancetta to a small plate, leaving the rendered fat in the pan.

2. Return the pan to medium-high heat. Add the brussels sprouts and stir to coat with the fat. Spread the brussels sprouts in an even layer and cook, undisturbed, until they begin to caramelize, 3 to 4 minutes. Add the remaining 1 tablespoon of oil and stir to combine. Continue to cook, without stirring, until the sprouts are completely soft and browned at the edges, 3 to 4 more minutes.

3. In a small bowl, stir together the lemon juice, vinegar, and maple syrup. Stir the mixture into the pan along with the pancetta and salt and pepper to taste. Mix well and make sure to scrape up any brown bits from the bottom of the pan. Remove from the heat and serve immediately.

Better Than Your Mom's Meatloaf
with Caramelized Onion Gravy

SERVES: 6 TO 8 | PREP: 30 MINUTES | COOK: 50 MINUTES | INACTIVE: 15 MINUTES

Most people probably wouldn't rate meatloaf as a top-ten meal, but they recognize it as an old-school staple in dinner rotations of the past. Let me change your mind with this contemporary take inspired by the one my mom made when I was growing up. It has a ton of flavor, and the gravy is something you might want to eat with a spoon!

FOR THE MEATLOAF

1 tablespoon extra-virgin olive oil

1 medium sweet onion such as Vidalia, finely chopped

3 medium carrots, finely chopped

1 tablespoon chopped garlic

1¾ teaspoons kosher salt

¼ teaspoon ground black pepper

¼ cup white wine

2 large eggs

2 tablespoons ketchup

2 tablespoons Dijon mustard

2 tablespoons Worcestershire sauce

1 cup panko bread crumbs

1 pound ground beef (I use 85% lean for meatloaf)

1 pound ground pork

¾ cup finely shredded mild Cheddar cheese

FOR THE CARAMELIZED ONION GRAVY

3 tablespoons unsalted butter

2 sweet onions such as Vidalia, sliced into ¼-inch half moons

1 teaspoon sugar

½ teaspoon kosher salt, plus more as needed

2 teaspoons balsamic vinegar

2 tablespoons all-purpose flour

2 cups reduced-sodium chicken broth

½ cup heavy cream

1 sprig fresh rosemary

1. **MAKE THE MEATLOAF:** Preheat the oven to 400°F. Line a large rimmed baking sheet with parchment paper.

2. In a medium skillet over medium heat, warm the oil. Add the onion and carrots and sauté, stirring occasionally, until they soften, 5 minutes. Add the garlic, ¼ teaspoon of the salt, and the pepper, and continue to sauté until the carrots are softened and the onion is translucent, 2 to 3 minutes.

3. Add the wine and bring to a simmer. Cook until most of the liquid has cooked away, about 3 minutes. Remove the pan from the heat and cool completely.

4. In a large bowl, whisk together the eggs, ketchup, mustard, and Worcestershire sauce. Stir in the panko, cooled vegetable mixture, and the remaining 1½ teaspoons of salt. Add the ground beef, ground pork, and cheese. Using your hands, mix to fully combine.

5. Divide the meat mixture in half and shape two loaves on the prepared pan, each about 9 by 3½ inches.

6. Bake until the meatloaves are lightly browned and a thermometer registers 160°F when inserted in the center, 40 to 45 minutes.

7. Meanwhile, **MAKE THE GRAVY:** In a large sauté pan over medium-low heat, melt the butter. Add the onions, stirring to coat them with butter. Cook gently, stirring often, until they are completely soft, about 10 minutes. Stir in the sugar and salt and continue to cook, stirring occasionally, until the onions begin to take on color, 10 to 12 minutes more.

8. Increase the heat to medium and stir the vinegar into the onions. Continue to cook, stirring often, until the onions are a deep, rich tawny brown, 15 to 18 minutes more.

CONTINUED ON PAGE 161

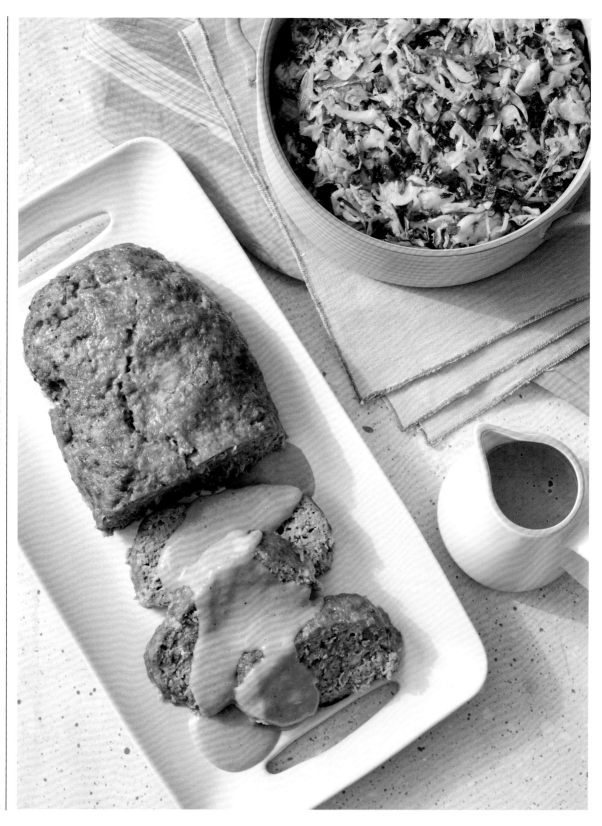

9. Sprinkle the flour over the onions, then stir in and cook 1 minute. Add the chicken broth and stir to combine. Continue cooking, stirring often, until the mixture thickens, 5 to 6 minutes. Stir in the cream and rosemary sprig and simmer to thicken slightly, 3 to 4 minutes.

10. Remove and discard the rosemary. Let the mixture cool for about 5 minutes, then carefully transfer to a blender and blend until smooth.

11. When the meatloaves are cooked, remove the pan from the oven and tent it with aluminum foil. Let rest for 15 minutes. While it rests, return the pureed gravy to the pan and simmer until heated through, 4 to 5 minutes. Season with salt to taste.

12. To serve, slice the meatloaves to the desired thickness and pass the gravy separately.

Balsamic Braised Beef Stew

SERVES: 4 TO 6 | PREP: 20 MINUTES | COOK: 2 HOURS 30 MINUTES

If it's a snowy or rainy day, you can be certain this is what's on my stove. This recipe is the reason why I always have beef chuck in the freezer, ready to go. You may be surprised by the amount of vinegar, but the balsamic cuts through the richness and helps highlight each ingredient in this dish.

2 pounds boneless beef chuck, trimmed, cut in 1½-inch cubes

⅓ cup all-purpose flour

1½ teaspoons kosher salt, plus more to taste

1½ teaspoons ground black pepper, plus more to taste

2 tablespoons extra-virgin olive oil, plus more, as needed

1 large red onion, sliced into ⅛-inch half moons

1 cup dry red wine (I like to use Cabernet)

1½ cups beef broth

2 bay leaves

3 large carrots, cut into ¼-inch-thick rounds

¼ cup balsamic vinegar

1 tablespoon cornstarch

Baked potatoes, for serving

Chopped parsley, for garnish (optional)

1. With paper towels, pat the meat dry. In a large shallow bowl, stir together the flour, salt, and pepper. Dredge the beef in the flour mixture, coating evenly and shaking off any excess.

2. In a large Dutch oven or heavy-bottomed pot over medium-high heat, heat the oil. Working in batches so as not to overcrowd the pan, add the meat and brown well on all sides, 10 to 12 minutes per batch. As each batch is browned, transfer it to a plate. Add more oil to the pan as needed to cook the remaining meat.

3. Add the onions to the meat drippings in the pan. Cook over medium-high heat, stirring several times, until they begin to soften and take on color, about 4 minutes.

4. Add the wine, and using a wooden spoon, stir up any brown bits from the bottom of the pot. Simmer for 2 minutes and then stir in the beef broth and bay leaves. Return the meat and any accumulated juices to the pot.

5. Bring the stew to a simmer, cover, and reduce the heat to low. Cook gently, stirring periodically, until the meat is fork-tender, about 1½ hours.

6. Add the carrots, cover, and continue cooking until the carrots are tender, 25 to 30 minutes. Add salt and pepper to taste and remove the bay leaves.

7. In a small bowl, stir together the vinegar and cornstarch to make a slurry. Stir it into the pot and simmer, uncovered, until the sauce has thickened, about 10 minutes.

8. To serve, adjust the seasoning to taste. Spoon over baked potatoes and sprinkle with parsley (if using).

NOTE

I like to serve this over baked potatoes, but you can instead serve it over plain pasta or polenta.

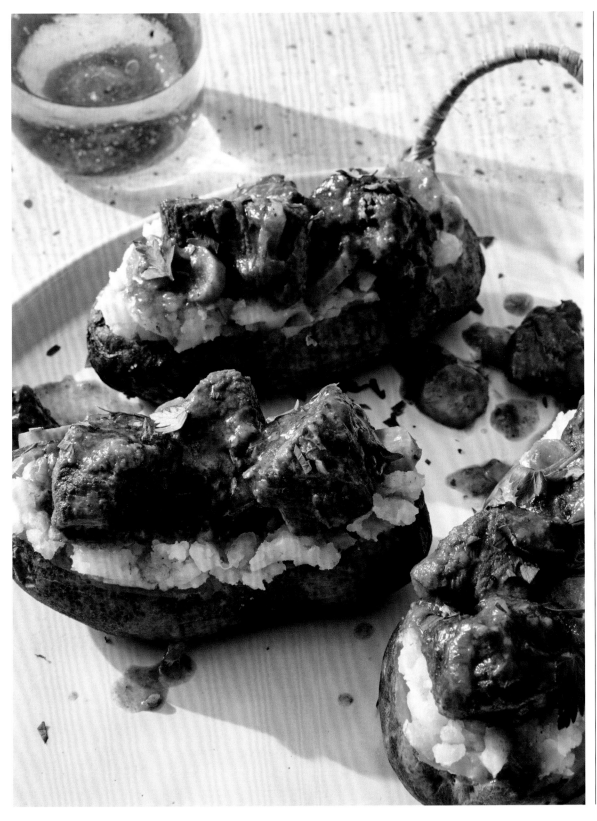

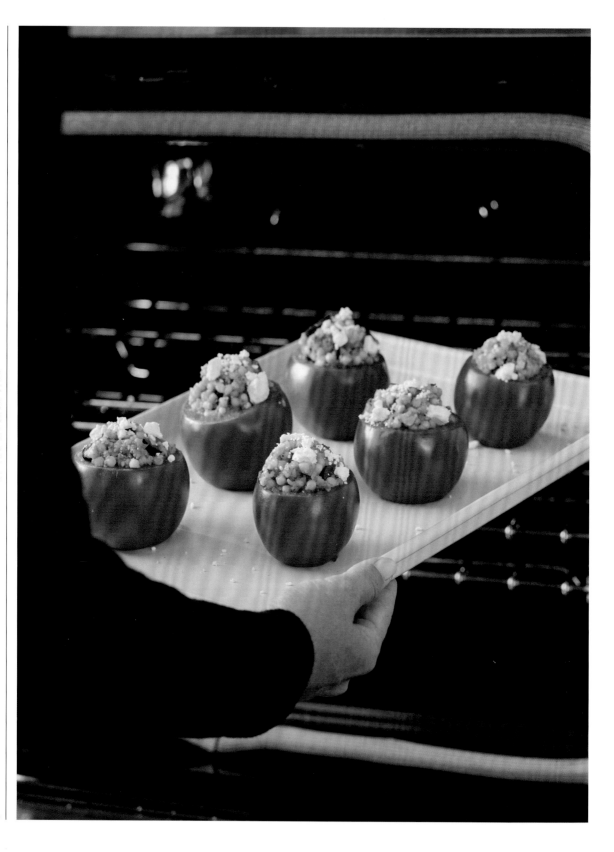

Mediterranean-Inspired Stuffed Tomatoes

SERVES: 6 | PREP: 20 MINUTES | COOK: 25 MINUTES

My love for tomatoes runs deep. I could eat them like apples, but I've found that stuffing them with couscous and olives and topping them with a bit of feta is an even better option. This is a great choice when you need a vegetarian main course or light, summery meal.

6 medium vine-ripened tomatoes

2 tablespoons extra-virgin olive oil, plus more for drizzling

1 tablespoon finely chopped garlic

⅓ cup chopped red onion

1 cup quick-cooking pearl couscous

½ cup chopped Kalamata olives

½ teaspoon kosher salt, plus more as needed

¼ teaspoon ground black pepper

¼ cup Italian-style bread crumbs

1½ tablespoons red wine vinegar

¼ teaspoon dried oregano

¼ cup crumbled feta cheese

Chopped fresh basil, for serving

MORE TO SHARE RECIPE

NOTE

To remove the pulp, it helps if you score the inside of the tomato with a knife, being careful not to pierce the flesh of the tomato. If you have a melon baller or serrated grapefruit spoon, they help make the task simple.

1. Preheat the oven to 400°F.

2. Slice off and discard the tops of the tomatoes. Using a spoon, carefully hollow out the tomatoes by removing the pulp and seeds, adding them to a medium bowl. As each tomato is hollowed out, place it upside down in a baking dish.

3. In a blender, blend the tomato seeds and pulp until smooth. Add water to reach the 2-cup line indicated on the blender jar; set aside.

4. Meanwhile, in a high-sided skillet over medium heat, warm the oil. Add the garlic and cook until fragrant, about 30 seconds. Add the onion and cook, stirring several times, until it begins to soften, about 2 minutes.

5. Add the couscous to the pan and toast, gently moving it around the pan for 1 minute. Stir in the tomato puree and bring to a gentle simmer. Add the olives, salt, and pepper and gently stir to combine.

6. Cover the pan and cook gently until the couscous is tender and has absorbed the liquid, 6 to 7 minutes. Remove from the heat and add the bread crumbs, vinegar, and oregano. Stir to combine.

7. Turn the tomatoes right-side up in the baking dish and lightly sprinkle the insides with salt. Divide the filling among the tomatoes, adding it until the couscous mixture reaches the top. Sprinkle feta cheese over the top of each tomato and drizzle with oil.

8. Bake the tomatoes, uncovered, until they have softened and the couscous filling is hot, about 15 minutes.

9. Sprinkle with basil and serve hot or at room temperature.

"Martha, Martha," the Lord answered, "you are worried and upset about many things, but few things are needed— or indeed only one. Mary has chosen what is better, and it will not be taken away from her."

LUKE 10:41–42

The story of Mary and Martha has always lived in the back of my mind, and I think about it often, especially when I'm tired or fed up.

I've always felt for Martha, in particular. Mary is the heroine in the story, praised for doing the right thing by sitting at Jesus's feet instead of busying herself preparing dinner and making sure the beds are made. Growing up, I understood the premise. Mary chose to sit and listen to the Lord instead of worrying about the state of the house. Listening to the words of the Lord was far more valuable. But it never sat completely right with me. I mean, who would be the hero when it was time for a snack—am I right?!

In this self-care-obsessed world, the Marthas can feel out of place, stuck between wanting to do good and overdoing it. I love hosting family and friends for dinner and being the go-to person when someone needs their kids watched last minute.

I like feeling dependable, although there is a darker side to it all. I find myself unable to sleep, trying to figure out how I will get it all done. Or I lean in to my empathetic side so much that I truly believe things will fall apart without me. Or I hold on to resentment because I said yes to something I shouldn't have. You might want to turn around yourself and yell, like Martha did, "Hey, Jesus, can you tell someone else to pitch in?!"

Yikes.

How do we find the right balance between Martha and Mary? Sometimes you need to bargain with yourself. Are you like me, and can't stand to *not* cook dinner? Turn on the slow cooker, and then sit down and read a book. You will still feed your family, yet you will be able to rest instead of actively cook. God has taught me that he wants me to catch a break. That

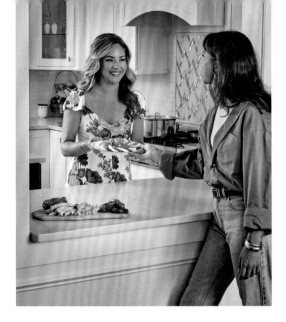

it doesn't all have to fall on my shoulders. He doesn't want me to get to the point where an illness needs to knock me off my feet. But hey, I am not a fast learner.

> Come to me, all you who are weary and burdened, and I will give you rest. Take my yoke upon you and learn from me, for I am gentle and humble in heart, and you will find rest for your souls. For my yoke is easy and my burden is light.
>
> MATTHEW 11:28–30

God loves the Marthas and Marys equally. Make sure you protect your servant's heart by using discernment and recognizing the need for rest. For the sake of enjoying today, separate the details that are important in the moment from those that can wait until tomorrow. Let God refresh you and include him in your decisions as you go about your day. Ask him to help you be present in the moments where he has truly called you to serve.

Dear Lord, thank you for equipping me with the tools and talents to serve. I pray you will give me discernment daily and help me be slow to overcommit and even slower to anger. Help me to know that rest is necessary and in obedience to you just as much as service. I pray you would raise up others in my absence.

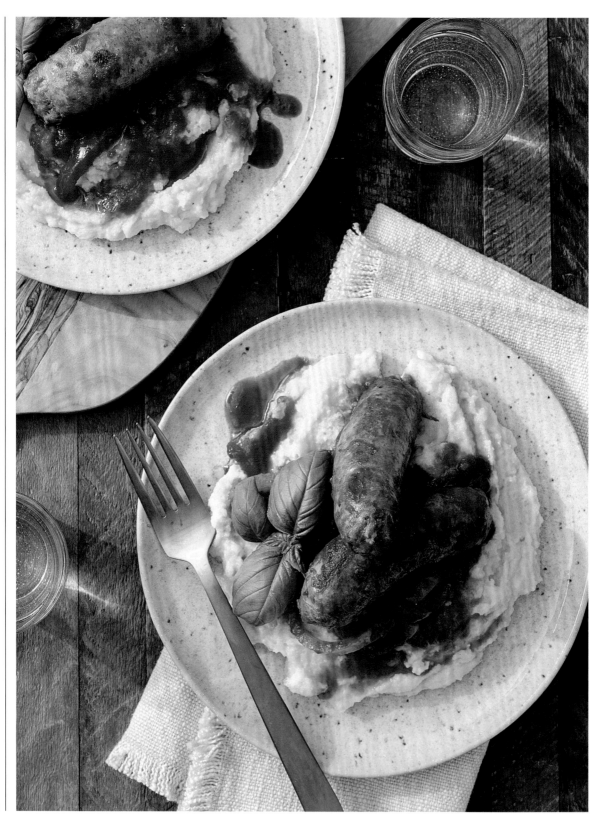

Sausage and Peppers
Over Creamy Polenta

SERVES: 3 TO 4 | PREP: 20 MINUTES | COOK: 45 MINUTES

Sausage and peppers are a favorite staple in my meal rotation, a winning recipe to serve on game days, lazy Sundays, and throughout barbecue season. I brought the two ideas together for a shortcut when you don't want to spend all day making your Sunday sauce.

FOR THE SAUSAGE AND PEPPERS

1 large red bell pepper, seeds and membranes removed, cut into ¼-inch slices

1 large yellow bell pepper, seeds and membranes removed, cut into ¼-inch slices

1 large sweet onion, such as Vidalia, cut in ¼-inch juliennes

¼ teaspoon kosher salt, plus more as needed

¼ teaspoon ground black pepper, plus more as needed

2½ teaspoons balsamic vinegar

3 tablespoons extra-virgin olive oil

2 large garlic cloves, crushed

1 pound (4 to 6 links) sweet Italian sausage, skin pierced with a knife

2 cups canned crushed tomatoes

6 leaves fresh basil, chiffonade, plus more for garnish

FOR THE CREAMY POLENTA

1½ teaspoons kosher salt, plus more as needed

2 cups instant polenta

½ cup heavy cream

2 tablespoons unsalted butter, room temperature

¼ cup plus 2 tablespoons freshly grated Parmigiano-Reggiano cheese

1. **MAKE THE SAUSAGE AND PEPPERS:** In a medium bowl, stir the red and yellow bell peppers, onion, salt, pepper, and 1 teaspoon of the vinegar to combine. Set aside.

2. In a large high-sided skillet over medium heat, warm the oil. Add the garlic and cook until soft and fragrant, 1 to 2 minutes. Add the sausage links and cook until well browned on all sides, about 12 minutes. Using tongs or a slotted spoon, remove and discard the garlic and transfer the sausages to a plate.

3. Add the pepper and onion mixture to the skillet and cook, stirring often, until the vegetables are soft and the onions begin to color, about 12 minutes.

4. Add the crushed tomatoes and ⅓ cup of water to the skillet and stir to combine. Bring to a gentle simmer, then stir in the remaining 1½ teaspoons vinegar and salt and pepper to taste. Nestle the sausages into the sauce; cover and cook until the sausages are cooked through, about 15 minutes. Remove from the heat and stir in the basil.

5. **MAKE THE CREAMY POLENTA:** In a medium saucepan, bring 5 cups cold water and 1½ teaspoons of the salt to a boil. Stirring constantly, add the polenta in a slow, steady stream. Cook over medium-low heat, stirring constantly, until the polenta thickens and starts to pull away from the sides of the pan, 4 to 8 minutes (or follow package instructions).

6. Add the cream, mix well, and then add the butter. Cook, stirring constantly, until it is melted and fully incorporated. Remove from the heat, stir in the cheese, and add salt to taste.

7. Divide the polenta among serving bowls. Top with a portion of the sausage and peppers, being sure to spoon some of the sauce over the top. Garnish with basil and serve immediately.

Fall French Onion Chicken

SERVES: 4 | PREP: 15 MINUTES | COOK: 1 HOUR 10 MINUTES

If you can't get enough French onion soup, this recipe is for you. Hang in there with caramelizing the onions—it's the longest part of the recipe but the most crucial. This has become a family favorite on those chillier nights. You can also make this earlier in the day if you hold off doing the last two steps until you are ready to eat.

FOR THE ONIONS

2 large yellow onions, thinly sliced into half moons

4 tablespoons (½ stick) unsalted butter

½ teaspoon kosher salt

1 teaspoon sugar

2 teaspoons balsamic vinegar

FOR THE CHICKEN

¼ cup all-purpose flour

1½ teaspoons kosher salt

¼ teaspoon ground black pepper

4 boneless, skinless chicken breasts

2 tablespoons extra-virgin olive oil

½ cup dry white wine

2 tablespoons dry sherry

1½ cups beef broth

2 sprigs fresh thyme

1 bay leaf

1 cup shredded Gruyère cheese

1. **MAKE THE ONIONS:** In a large Dutch oven or enameled cast-iron braiser over low heat, melt the butter. Add the onions and cook undisturbed for 10 minutes. Sprinkle the salt over the onions and gently stir to combine. Cook without stirring for 10 minutes. Stir in the sugar and vinegar and continue to cook, stirring periodically, until the onions are a rich caramel color, about 25 minutes more. Transfer them to a bowl and set aside. Set the pot aside to use for the chicken.

2. Meanwhile, **MAKE THE CHICKEN:** In a large shallow bowl, whisk together the flour, ½ teaspoon salt, and ⅛ teaspoon pepper. Dredge the chicken breasts in the seasoned flour, fully coating both sides and shaking off any excess.

3. Return the pot to medium-high heat and add the oil. When it is hot, add the chicken breasts and cook, turning once, until golden brown on each side, about 6 minutes per side. Transfer the cooked chicken to a large plate.

4. With the pot over medium-high heat, pour in the wine and sherry. Using a wooden spoon, stir to loosen any browned bits from the bottom of the pan. Return the onions to the pan, bring to a simmer, and cook for 3 minutes.

5. Add the beef broth, thyme, bay leaf, the remaining 1 teaspoon salt, and ⅛ teaspoon pepper and stir to combine. Add the chicken and any accumulated juice, nestling the chicken into the onions. Cover and simmer until the chicken is cooked through, 12 to 15 minutes. Remove the pan from the heat.

6. Carefully remove the lid and sprinkle the cheese evenly over the chicken. Place under a heated broiler and broil, watching closely, until the cheese begins to bubble and brown, about 5 minutes. Serve immediately.

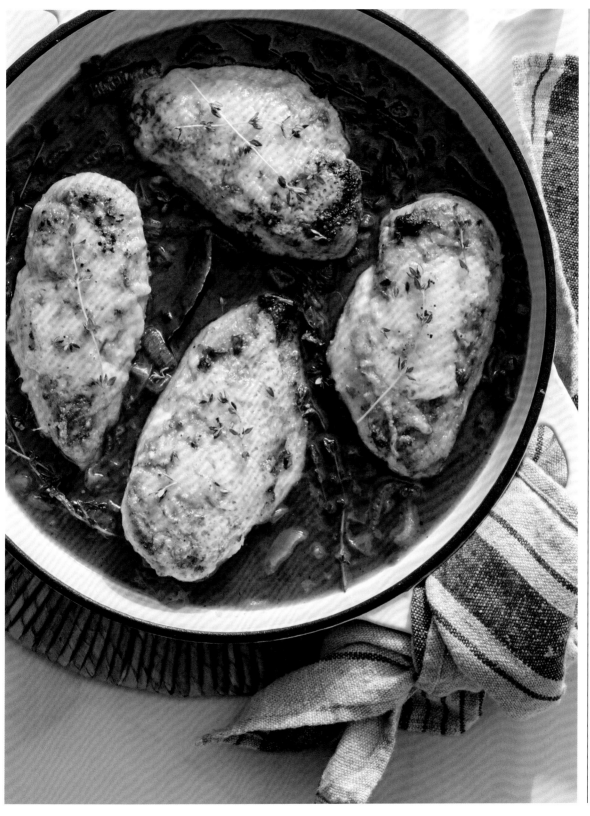

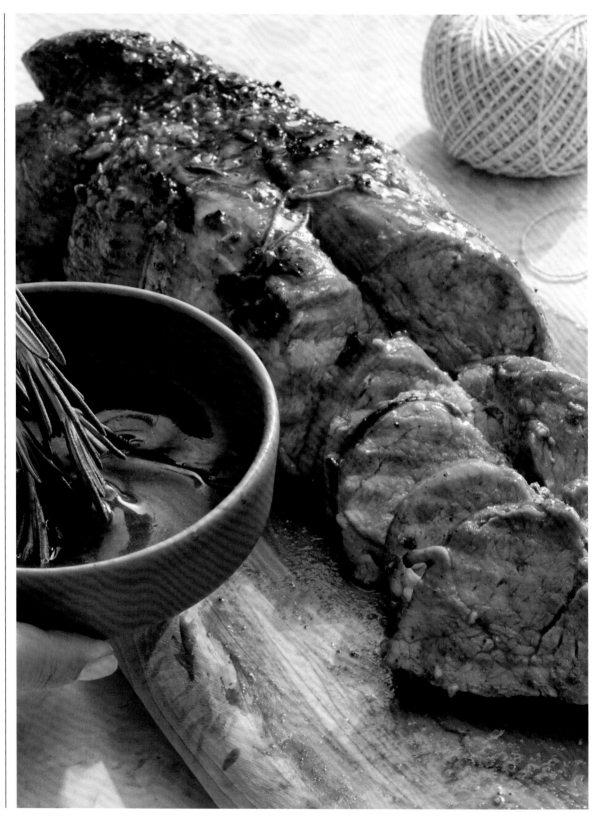

Brown Sugar Pork Tenderloin

SERVES: 4 TO 6 | PREP: 15 MINUTES | COOK: 40 MINUTES | INACTIVE: 1 HOUR 40 MINUTES

To be honest, I served this pork dish to Siena, telling her it was chicken. I'm not proud of lying, but I knew she would love it if I could get her to try it. We do what we have to, right? The recipe is a favorite among both kids and adults. You can marinate the pork earlier in the day and then pop it in the oven prior to dinnertime. I love to use pork loin when entertaining because it serves a group of people, while only requiring me to open and close the oven!

2 pounds boneless pork tenderloin

Kosher salt

Ground black pepper

¼ cup packed light brown sugar

2 tablespoons Dijon mustard

1 tablespoon extra-virgin olive oil

1 tablespoon minced garlic

1½ teaspoons chopped fresh rosemary

1 teaspoon smoked paprika

¼ cup dry sherry

1. Place the pork in a 9 by 13-inch glass or ceramic baking dish. Using the tines of a fork and working down the length of the tenderloin, pierce the meat about ¼-inch deep. Generously season all sides with salt and pepper.

2. In a small bowl, mix together the brown sugar, mustard, oil, garlic, rosemary, paprika, and salt and pepper, to taste, to make a paste. Rub the mixture all over the pork loin until well coated. Cover the pan and marinate in the refrigerator for at least 30 minutes or up to 8 hours. Remove it from the refrigerator 1 hour before baking to allow it to come to room temperature.

3. Preheat the oven to 400°F.

4. Pour the sherry around the pork in the bottom of the baking dish. Bake, uncovered, until the meat registers 145°F at the thickest part, about 30 minutes.

5. Transfer the pork to a cutting board, ideally with a trench to collect the juices. Cover with aluminum foil and let rest for 10 minutes.

6. To serve, slice the pork to the desired thickness and transfer to a serving platter. Pour any accumulated juices from the cutting board into the baking dish and stir together, then spoon over the sliced meat.

Butternut Squash Lasagna
with Sage and Goat Cheese

SERVES: 6 | PREP: 45 MINUTES | COOK: 1 HOUR 45 MINUTES | INACTIVE: 30 MINUTES

This lasagna is a labor of love, partially because everyone you serve it to will instantly love you. This lasagna has won me accolades within my family and helped me win the Best Home Cook Contest on Hallmark Channel's *Home & Family*. It's also a great option for family and friends who prefer not to eat meat.

FOR THE SQUASH

1 small (about 1 pound) butternut
   squash, halved lengthwise and seeded

2½ tablespoons extra-virgin olive oil

4 sprigs fresh thyme

2 unpeeled garlic cloves

Kosher salt

Ground black pepper

FOR THE LASAGNA

Kosher salt

1 (1-pound) package lasagna noodles

5 tablespoons unsalted butter

3 fresh sage leaves

¼ cup all-purpose flour

3 cups whole milk

1 cup grated pecorino Romano cheese

1¼ cups crumbled goat cheese

¼ teaspoon nutmeg

⅛ teaspoon ground black pepper

FOR THE BREAD CRUMB TOPPING

½ cup panko bread crumbs

2 tablespoons unsalted butter, melted

1½ teaspoons chopped fresh sage

2 teaspoons fresh thyme leaves

½ teaspoon kosher salt

MORE TO SHARE RECIPE

1. **PREPARE THE SQUASH:** Preheat the oven to 425°F. Line a rimmed baking sheet with aluminum foil.

2. Place the squash, cut-side up, on the prepared baking sheet and drizzle with oil. Place 2 sprigs of thyme and 1 garlic clove in each cavity and season with salt and pepper.

3. Bake the squash until it is browned in spots and fork-tender, about 50 minutes. Remove from the oven and let cool until it can be easily handled, about 20 minutes. Remove and discard the thyme sprigs. Peel the garlic cloves and place them in a large bowl.

4. Reduce the oven temperature to 375°F.

5. Scoop the flesh from the squash and add it to the bowl with the garlic. Season with ½ teaspoon salt and ¼ teaspoon pepper. Using a hand mixer or immersion blender, mix the squash on low speed until it is completely smooth.

6. **MAKE THE LASAGNA:** Bring a large pot of water to a boil. Add 1 tablespoon of salt and the lasagna noodles. Cook until the noodles are al dente, using the package directions for suggested timing. Drain, reserving ½ cup of the pasta cooking water. Immediately arrange the noodles in a single layer on a large cloth to prevent them from sticking together.

7. In a medium saucepan over medium-high heat, melt the butter. Add the sage leaves and cook until they're fragrant, about 2 minutes. Remove and discard the sage.

8. Reduce the heat to low and whisk in the flour. Cook, whisking constantly, until the mixture turns a pale tan color, 6 to 7 minutes. Whisking constantly, slowly add the milk.

CONTINUED ON PAGE 177

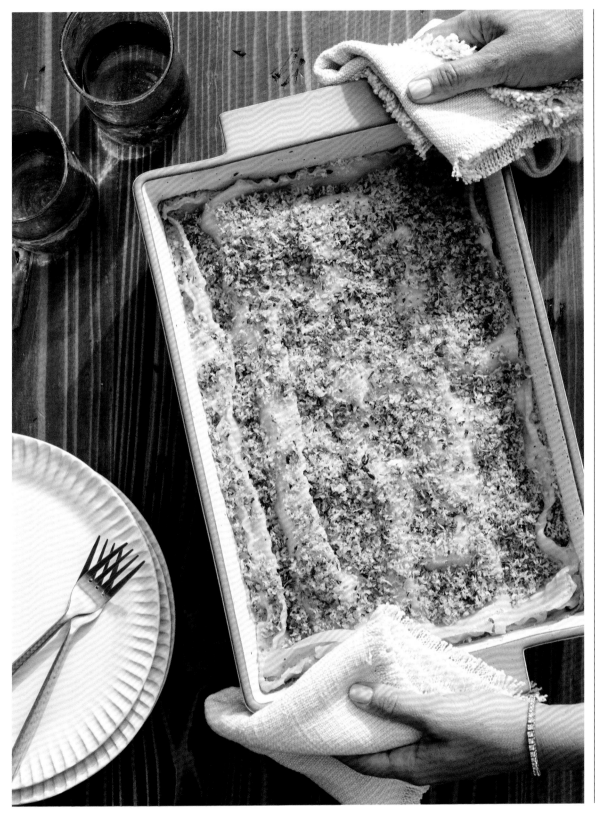

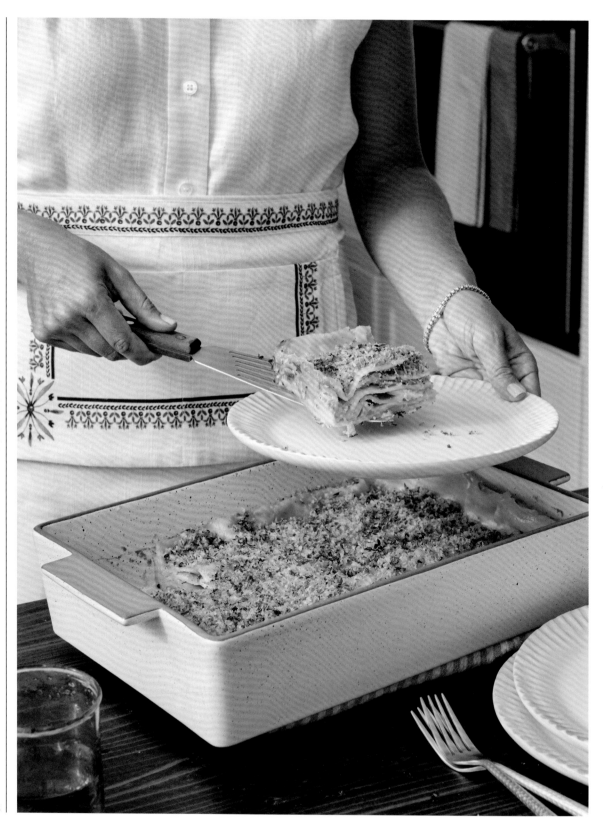

9. Bring the mixture to a simmer and cook, stirring occasionally and scraping the bottom and sides of the pan, until the sauce has thickened and coats the back of a spoon, 10 to 12 minutes. Remove the pan from the heat and add ½ cup of the pecorino Romano, the goat cheese, nutmeg, 1 teaspoon of salt, and pepper and stir until smooth.

10. Measure out and set aside 1½ cups of the cheese sauce. Stir the remaining sauce into the squash mixture.

11. **MAKE THE BREAD CRUMB TOPPING:** In a medium bowl, mix the panko, butter, sage, thyme, and salt until well combined.

12. To assemble the lasagna, spread half of the reserved sauce over the bottom of a 9 by 13-inch baking dish. Add a layer of the lasagna noodles, overlapping them slightly to cover the entire bottom. Spread 1 cup of the squash mixture evenly over the noodles. Repeat the layering of noodles and squash mixture three more times, finishing with a layer of noodles.

13. Whisk the reserved pasta cooking water into the remaining cheese sauce. Pour evenly over the top noodle layer, then sprinkle with the bread crumb topping and then the remaining ½ cup of pecorino Romano cheese.

14. Cover the pan with aluminum foil and bake for 40 minutes. Remove the foil and bake, uncovered, until the lasagna is hot in the center and the top is lightly browned, about 15 minutes more. Remove from the oven and let stand for 10 minutes before serving.

Baked Penne Vodka

SERVES: 4 TO 6 | PREP: 20 MINUTES | COOK: 40 MINUTES

I'm sent into a tailspin whenever someone asks, "What's your favorite thing to make?" There are so many foods that I enjoy prepping, sharing, and consuming! However, this Baked Penne Vodka has become my top answer. It is one of the few recipes I thought about not sharing online when I first dreamed of having a book.

Kosher salt

1 (16-ounce) box penne pasta

1 (8-ounce) piece low-moisture whole milk mozzarella cheese

2 tablespoons extra-virgin olive oil

2 tablespoons minced garlic

1 teaspoon crushed red pepper flakes

1 (28-ounce) can crushed tomatoes

1 teaspoon freshly ground black pepper

¾ cup vodka

4 tablespoons (½ stick) unsalted butter

½ cup heavy cream

½ cup fresh basil, roughly chopped

¼ cup mascarpone cheese

3 cups fresh baby spinach, coarsely chopped

½ cup freshly grated pecorino Romano cheese

NOTE

Garnish with fresh basil leaves, if you have some on hand.

MORE TO SHARE RECIPE

1. Preheat the oven to 375°F.

2. Bring a large pot of water to a boil. Add 1 tablespoon of salt and the pasta. Cook until al dente, 8 to 10 minutes. Drain well and set aside.

3. Meanwhile, cut six ¼-inch-thick slices from the piece of mozzarella and grate the remainder using the large holes of a box grater; set aside.

4. In a medium high-sided pan over medium-high heat, warm the oil. Add the garlic and red pepper flakes and cook, stirring several times, until fragrant, about 1 minute.

5. Stir in the tomatoes, 1¼ teaspoons of salt, and the pepper. Bring to a simmer and cook, stirring often, until the tomatoes have thickened slightly, 4 to 5 minutes. Add the vodka and continue to simmer until the sauce coats the back of a wooden spoon, 6 to 7 minutes. Stir in the butter. When it has fully melted, add the cream and basil, stirring constantly as you do so. Simmer 2 to 3 minutes to combine the flavors, then remove the pan from the heat.

6. Off the heat, add the mascarpone, stirring gently until it is fully melted into the sauce, and then fold in the spinach.

7. Spread ¼ cup of the tomato sauce over the bottom of a 9 by 13-inch baking dish. Add half of the pasta and then half of the remaining tomato sauce, spooning it so that all the pasta is covered with sauce. Repeat with another layer of pasta and then the remaining sauce.

8. Arrange the sliced mozzarella over the pasta, then use the shredded mozzarella to fill any gaps. Sprinkle the pecorino Romano evenly over the top.

9. Cover the pan with aluminum foil and bake for 10 minutes. Remove the foil and bake until the pasta is hot throughout and the cheese begins to bubble, about 15 minutes. Serve immediately.

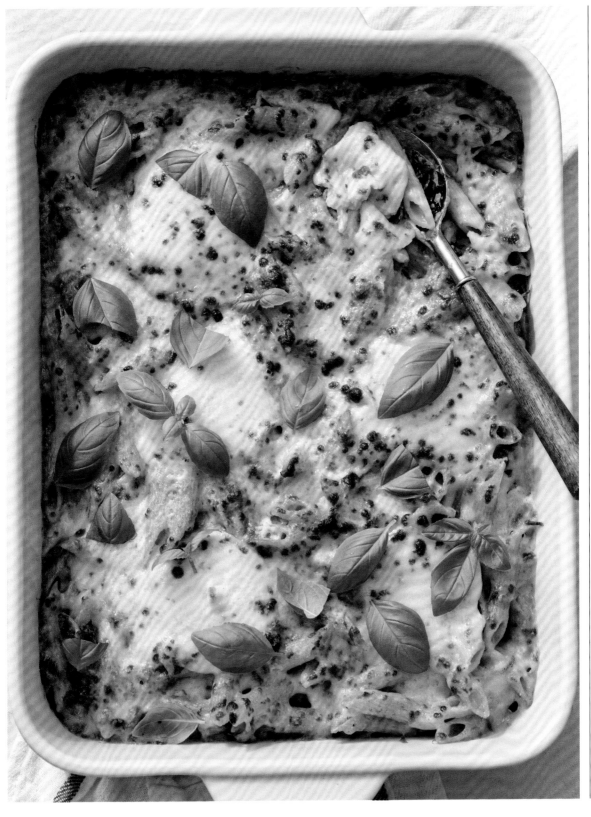

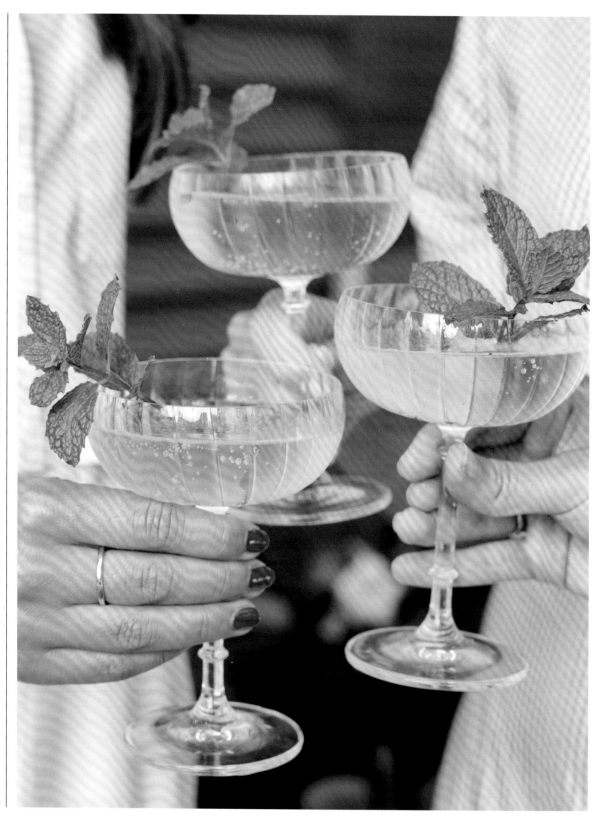

Big Batch Hugo Spritz

SERVES: 8 TO 10 | PREP: 5 MINUTES

One year, my friends and I took a dream trip to Italy. I almost missed out because of my last-minute realization that my passport had expired—but the important part is I made it. In Italy, I proceeded to drink many Hugo Spritzes while braving the extremely hot and humid Sorrento sun.

1 (2-liter) bottle soda water, chilled

1 (750 ml) bottle prosecco, chilled

1 cup elderflower liqueur (I like St. Germain), chilled

½ cup Mint Simple Syrup (page 217), chilled

Fresh mint, for serving (optional)

Lime wedges, for serving (optional)

1. In a large pitcher, gently stir the soda water, prosecco, elderflower liqueur, and simple syrup to combine.

2. Pour into wine glasses and serve immediately with a garnish of mint leaves or lime wedge (if using).

NOTE

Freeze some lime slices and add them to the pitcher to help keep the drink cool!

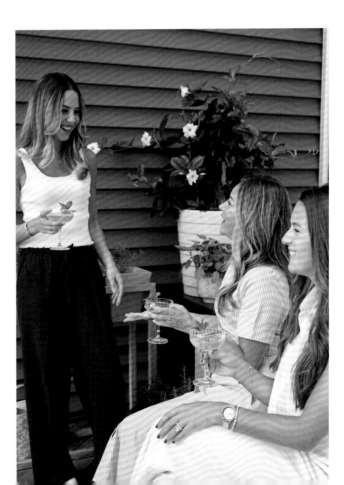

Crispy Eggplant Stacks
with Olive Tapenade

SERVES: 6 | PREP: 25 MINUTES | COOK: 15 MINUTES | INACTIVE: 10 MINUTES

This is one of those dishes that's easy enough for a weeknight but looks impressive enough for a dinner party. The eggplant comes out super crispy thanks to the panko, and the olive tapenade is not only great in this dish but works well on sandwiches or folded into warm pasta. It also makes a great addition to a cheese and crackers board!

FOR THE OLIVE TAPENADE

1 cup pitted oil-cured olives

¼ cup extra-virgin olive oil

1 garlic clove, chopped

1 tablespoon chopped fresh basil

FOR THE EGGPLANT

1 medium eggplant, peeled and sliced into thin rounds (about ⅛ inch)

2 large eggs

1 cup panko bread crumbs

½ cup all-purpose flour

½ teaspoon garlic powder

½ teaspoon dried basil

½ teaspoon kosher salt, plus more as needed

¼ cup extra-virgin olive oil, plus more as needed

1 large beefsteak tomato, cut in ¼-inch-thick slices

1 large (8-ounce) ball fresh mozzarella cheese, cut in ¼-inch slices

Balsamic glaze, for serving

Chopped fresh basil, for serving

NOTE

You can find oil-cured olives on most olive bars. Other olives, such as Kalamata olives or black olives, would work, although the flavor will be different.

1. **MAKE THE TAPENADE:** In a mini food processor, pulse the olives, oil, and garlic to uniformly chop the olives. They should be a little chunky but fine enough to spread. They also can be finely minced by hand. Transfer to a small bowl and stir in the basil.

2. **MAKE THE EGGPLANT:** Place the eggplant slices in a large bowl, cover with cold water, and let soak for 10 minutes.

3. In the meantime, set up a dredging station. Lightly whisk the eggs in a large shallow bowl. In another shallow bowl, stir together the panko, flour, garlic powder, basil, and salt.

4. Drain the eggplant and pat dry with a paper towel. Dip each slice in the eggs, coating both sides and letting the excess drip off. Dip the slices in the panko mixture, turning to fully coat both sides and gently patting the crumbs in place. Arrange the coated slices on a baking sheet.

5. In a large sauté pan over medium-high heat, warm ¼ cup of the oil until a few panko crumbs sizzle when added. Fry the eggplant in batches, adding a single layer to the hot oil. Cook, turning once, until crisp and golden on both sides, about 2 minutes per side. Transfer to a paper towel–lined plate as they are cooked and sprinkle lightly with salt. Fry the remaining eggplant, adding more oil as needed.

6. To assemble the stacks, place one slice of the eggplant on a serving plate and top with a slice of tomato. Spread 1 tablespoon of the tapenade on the tomato. Continue layering as follows: mozzarella slice, eggplant slice, and 1 tablespoon of tapenade. Garnish with a drizzle of balsamic glaze and a sprinkle of basil.

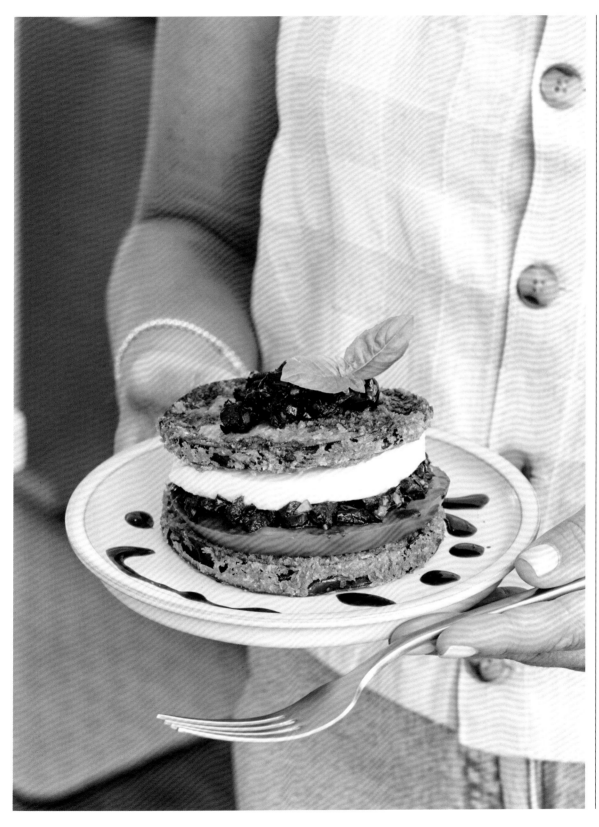

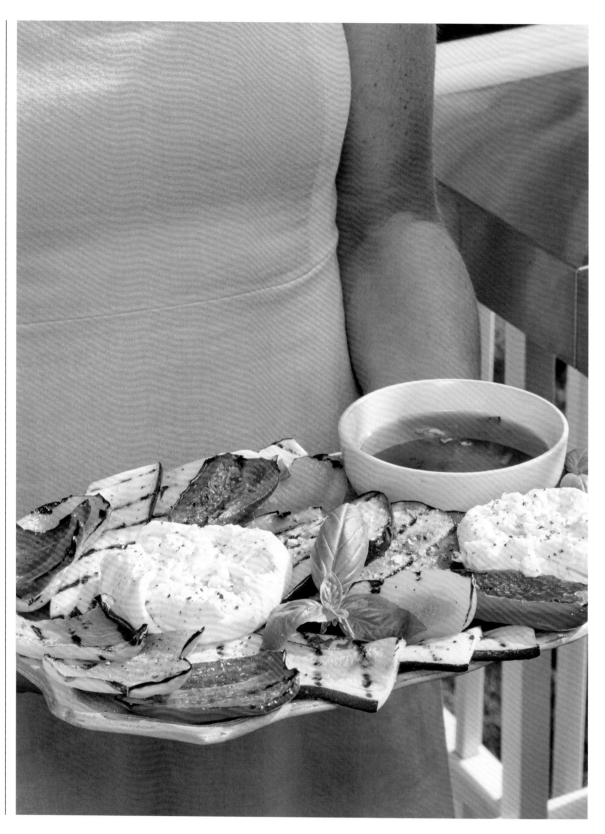

Grilled Vegetables
with Lemon Basil Vinaigrette

SERVES: 4 TO 6 | PREP: 20 MINUTES | COOK: 15 MINUTES | INACTIVE: 20 MINUTES

This dish gets bonus points for beauty. The colorful veggies with grill marks make for an impressive presentation. It's the perfect side for summer meals.

FOR THE VINAIGRETTE

½ cup extra-virgin olive oil

½ cup fresh basil leaves, chopped

2 tablespoons freshly squeezed lemon juice

2 garlic cloves, minced

½ teaspoon plus a pinch of kosher salt

⅛ teaspoon ground black pepper

FOR THE VEGETABLES

1 large unpeeled eggplant, sliced into ¼-inch rounds

2 medium zucchini, sliced lengthwise into ¼-inch-thick slices

1 teaspoon kosher salt

2 red bell peppers, cored, quartered, and seeds removed

2 yellow bell peppers, cored, quartered, and seeds removed

2 (4-ounce) balls burrata cheese, drained

1. **MAKE THE VINAIGRETTE:** In a small bowl, whisk together the oil, basil, lemon juice, garlic, salt, and pepper.

2. **MAKE THE VEGETABLES:** In a colander set over a bowl, combine the eggplant and zucchini slices, sprinkle with the salt, and toss gently to combine; let drain for 20 minutes. Pat the slices dry with paper towels and place in a large bowl. Discard the accumulated liquid.

3. Add the bell peppers and ¼ cup of the vinaigrette to the bowl and gently toss to coat.

4. Meanwhile, preheat a grill to 350°F.

5. Place the vegetables crosswise on the grates, close the lid, and cook, turning once or twice, until the vegetables are tender, about 4 minutes per side for the eggplant and zucchini, and about 6 minutes per side for the bell peppers.

6. To serve, arrange the grilled vegetables on a serving platter and brush lightly with the vinaigrette. Gently break the burrata to expose the centers and rest them over the vegetables. Serve hot or at room temperature.

NOTE

The vinaigrette makes more than you need. It can be refrigerated for up to 5 days. Use it to dress a simple salad or as a marinade.

You also can serve the burrata on the side of this dish, letting people add the cheese as desired.

Saucy Baby Back Ribs

SERVES: 4 | PREP: 20 MINUTES | COOK: 2 HOURS 45 MINUTES | INACTIVE: 1 HOUR 20 MINUTES

These ribs have earned me rave reviews across the board. Even friends from down south have commented that they are some of the best they've ever had. I am not saying I am a pit master, but I am proud of this recipe. Besides the cooking method, the Chinese five spice powder in the rub and sauce is the secret weapon. Well, not so secret anymore!

FOR THE RIBS

2 teaspoons smoked paprika

2 teaspoons kosher salt

2 teaspoons ground black pepper

1 teaspoon Chinese five spice powder

1 teaspoon ground mustard

1 teaspoon garlic powder

1 teaspoon onion powder

¼ teaspoon chipotle chili powder

1 (2-pound) rack pork loin back ribs

FOR THE BARBECUE SAUCE

1½ cups packed dark brown sugar

1½ cups ketchup

2 tablespoons apple cider vinegar

2 tablespoons Worcestershire sauce

1 tablespoon fresh orange juice

1 tablespoon soy sauce

1½ teaspoons kosher salt

1 teaspoon black pepper

½ teaspoon Chinese five spice powder

¼ teaspoon chipotle chili powder

NOTE

As they're baking, insert a toothpick into the middle of your ribs. If it goes through easily, that indicates that the ribs are tender.

Any remaining sauce can be refrigerated in an airtight container for up to 2 weeks.

1. **MAKE THE RIBS:** In a small bowl, stir together the smoked paprika, salt, pepper, five spice powder, mustard, garlic powder, onion powder, and chili powder.

2. Place the ribs, curved-side up, on a large sheet of aluminum foil. Using a blunt knife, slide the rounded tip of the blade underneath the white membrane to loosen it to the point where you can easily grab it; then, using a paper towel, pull the membrane off the rack and discard. Blot the ribs dry with a paper towel.

3. Rub a generous coat of the spice mixture over both sides of the ribs. Tightly wrap the foil around the ribs and let marinate in the refrigerator for at least 1 hour. Remove them from the refrigerator 20 minutes before cooking.

4. Preheat the oven to 250°F.

5. Place the foil-wrapped ribs on a baking sheet and bake until the ribs are tender and the two center bones pull apart easily, about 2½ hours.

6. Meanwhile, **MAKE THE BARBECUE SAUCE:** In a medium pan, whisk together the brown sugar, ketchup, vinegar, Worcestershire sauce, orange juice, soy sauce, salt, pepper, five spice powder, and chipotle chili powder. Place the pan over medium heat and cook, stirring several times, until slightly thickened, 7 to 8 minutes. Set aside.

7. Preheat a grill to medium heat, 350°F.

8. Carefully unwrap the ribs and place them on a tray. Brush both sides of the ribs with a liberal coat of the sauce.

9. Place the ribs on the grill, close the cover, and cook for 7 minutes. Brush the top with sauce, then flip and brush the other side with sauce. Close the cover and cook for an additional 7 minutes. Serve immediately.

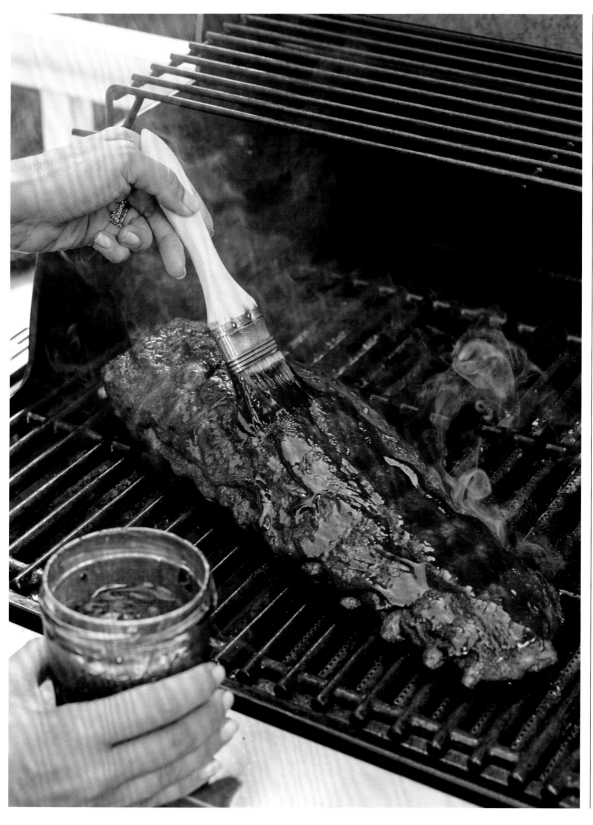

8

Can I Have a Treat?

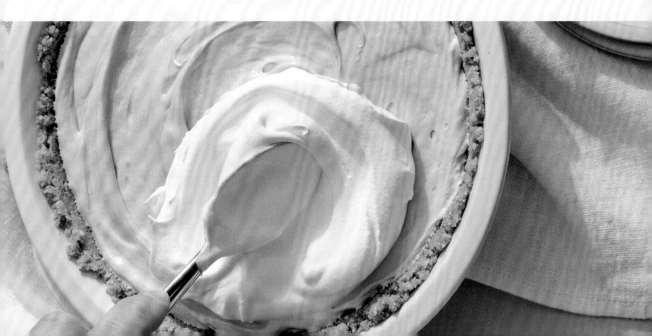

How truly sweet it is to be loved by a God who desires the best for us. His death on the cross so that we can have eternal life is more than we deserve. His love is unfailing, steadfast, and unchanging. He offers his promises for us to lean on and wants us to experience life in him to the fullest.

The joy of the Lord is not meant to be a fickle emotion. It can sustain us through both good and bad seasons of life. Learning to access and accept that joy can be the greatest blessing. When we can be grateful in any season and recognize God's goodness in the smallest details, then we can find the greatest level of contentment.

One of my favorite moments in hosting is when you set the dessert on the table. At that moment you are personally celebrating the finish line. Your guests are full and content, and you gladly cut yourself the largest piece of No-Bake Cookie Butter Pie (page 200). Alternatively, having the Cannoli Dip recipe (page 194) in your back pocket means you will never be without an easy sweet treat!

You know that feeling you get after a great meal? You settle back in your chair and feel your heart smile. My dream meal would be a great antipasto spread, followed by Baked Penne Vodka (page 178), and finishing with the Almond Trifle (page 203) from this chapter—all at Sunday dinner with my family. That is true contentment, right there!

Contentment is often a challenging and fleeting emotion. I have been through many long periods of discontentment. If I am honest, it creeps up on me more than I would like to admit. I mean how can it not? We are endlessly scrolling through social media, which constantly reminds us of what we don't have, what we could do better, and what we wish we could be. Before long, we start forgetting deep gratitude and contentment that once satisfied.

Have you ever wondered what it would have been like to grow up in our parents' time, before there was unlimited access to *all* the things? They didn't have a 24/7 newsfeed to compare their homes to. Even thinking back to teenage years, we had magazines to purchase and thumb through, but not continually updated altered images to scroll through until 3 A.M. No wonder contentment and joy have become more elusive. We work so hard to obtain status or material things that we think will make us happy, but they're only a temporary high that leaves us empty, wanting the next thing.

> I am not saying this because I am in need, for I have learned to be content whatever the circumstances. I know what it is to be in need, and I know what it is to have plenty. I have learned the secret of being content in any and every situation, whether well fed or hungry, whether living in plenty or in want. I can do all this through him who gives me strength.
>
> PHILIPPIANS 4:11–13

It is not that we should be void of desires or aspire to have nothing. God wants us to live a full and joyful life. However, checking the *why* behind our wants is sometimes a necessary exercise. When our desires cause frustration, bitterness, and constant unrest, it can be an indicator that they have become a nagging sin.

Contentment is usually found in simpler forms. It's when your child gives you that unexpected hug or lays their head on your shoulder, and you feel your heart swell. It's the calm you feel when you sit in your yard on a warm summer's evening, sharing laughter with friends. It's when you realize the rainy day on a weekend is just what you needed, and you settle in with a book and blanket, grateful for the quiet.

Does any of this stop us from wanting? Let's be honest: No, it does not. But we can learn to temper our expectations, putting those wants in perspective instead of letting them become all we see.

———————

Dear Lord, open my eyes to blessings that surround me daily. Help me be easily reminded of your goodness, not taking anything for granted. I do not want to miss what you have for me in the present moment. Help me to take time to sit in the good moments, instead of rushing to the next.

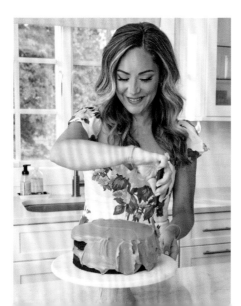

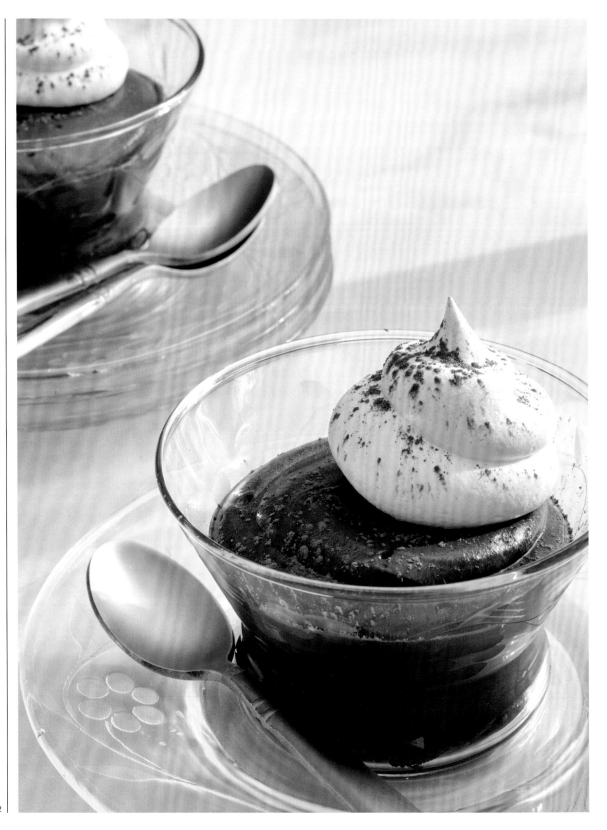

Spiced Chocolate Mousse

SERVES: 8 | PREP: 20 MINUTES | INACTIVE: 2 HOURS

When we first started dating, Brian and I occasionally took cooking classes. We both love food, so it was a fun way to spend time together and a great way for me to strengthen my culinary skills as well. Our first class together had this wonderful chocolate mousse that we couldn't forget! It's a classic preparation but super simple to make and a great make-ahead option. It feels to me like a grown-up version of pudding.

1½ cups chilled heavy cream

1⅔ cups sugar

1 large egg

2 large egg yolks

2 tablespoons brewed espresso, chilled

¼ teaspoon vanilla extract

⅛ teaspoon ground cinnamon

⅛ teaspoon ground nutmeg

⅛ teaspoon ground allspice

1¼ cups unsweetened cocoa powder, sifted

Quick Whip (page 216), for serving (optional)

1. In a medium bowl, use a hand mixer on medium speed to beat the cream and ⅓ cup of the sugar at medium speed until frothy. Sprinkle in another ⅓ cup of the sugar and continue to beat until stiff peaks form. Set aside in the refrigerator.

2. In a large bowl, use a hand mixer on high speed to beat the egg and egg yolks with the remaining 1 cup sugar until the mixture thickens and becomes pale yellow, 4 to 5 minutes. Add the espresso, vanilla, cinnamon, nutmeg, and allspice. Beat on low speed to combine, about 30 seconds.

3. Add the cocoa powder and beat on low until the mixture becomes very thick, 1 to 2 minutes.

4. Add about a third of the whipped cream and stir well to loosen and lighten the chocolate mixture. Spoon the remaining whipped cream on top. Using a flexible spatula, gently fold and turn it into the chocolate mixture, just until the cream disappears.

5. Divide the mousse among eight (6-ounce) ramekins or pudding dishes. Cover with plastic wrap and refrigerate for at least 2 hours, and up to 24 hours. Serve with Quick Whip (if using).

NOTE

Making this ahead of time allows the flavors to develop a bit more. It does not have to sit for 24 hours; making it 2 hours ahead of time is plenty of time as well!

Cannoli Dip

This is a top choice when I need something for a crowd or have impromptu guests. I started serving cannoli dip for game days, and it has since snuck into the regular rotation. The addition of cinnamon, although not traditional, along with the mascarpone, is my secret weapon for making the dip irresistible.

1 (15-ounce) container whole milk ricotta cheese

½ cup mascarpone cheese

½ teaspoon vanilla extract

Scant ⅛ teaspoon ground cinnamon

1 cup confectioners' sugar

¼ cup heavy cream

¾ cup mini chocolate chips

Vanilla pizzelle or other cookies, for serving

1. In a large mixing bowl, use a hand mixer on medium speed to whip the ricotta, mascarpone, vanilla, and cinnamon until well combined and smooth.

2. With the mixer on low, gradually add the sugar, beating well after each addition. Continue to beat until the mixture is fully combined and smooth.

3. Add the cream and beat on high speed until the mixture is silky and thickened, about 2 minutes. Do not overmix or the mixture will curdle.

4. Fold in the chocolate chips and transfer the mixture to a serving bowl. Serve with pizzelle or cookies of your choice.

NOTE

The dip can be made up to 2 days in advance and refrigerated. Stir gently before serving.

For a kid favorite, you also can serve the dip with broken pieces of waffle cones.

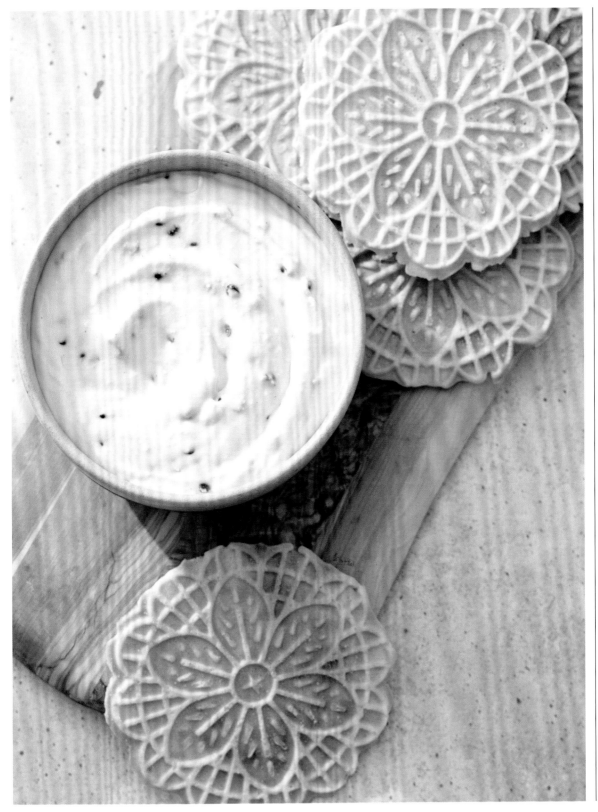

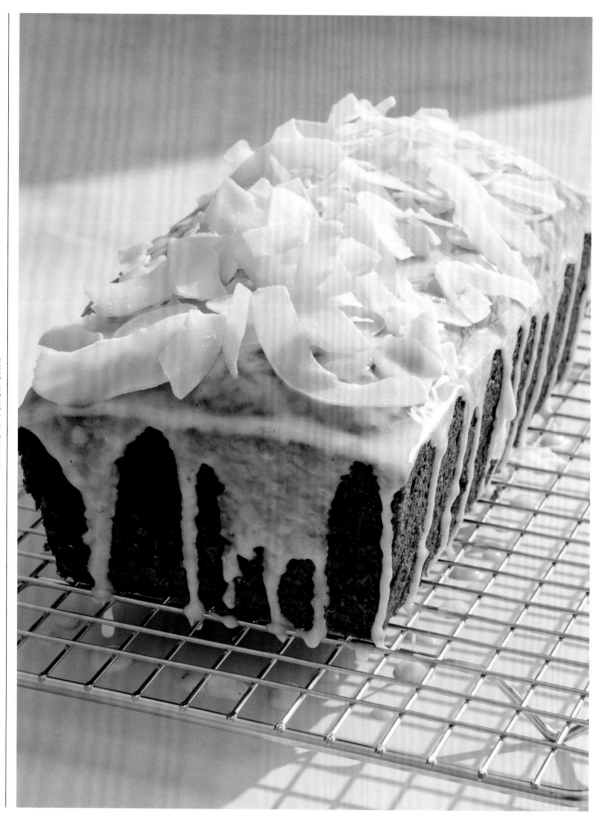

Pineapple Banana Bread

SERVES: 8 | PREP: 20 MINUTES | COOK: 50 MINUTES | INACTIVE: 1 HOUR

Ever feel like you can't make one more banana bread? I hear you, and I have been there. That's how this quick bread came to be. I was craving a tropical vacation in the middle of winter, and that desperation may or may not have turned to inspiration.

FOR THE BREAD

2 cups all-purpose flour

1 teaspoon baking powder

½ teaspoon baking soda

⅛ teaspoon salt

8 tablespoons (1 stick) unsalted butter, room temperature

½ cup granulated sugar

½ cup packed light brown sugar

2 large eggs, room temperature

1 ripe banana, mashed

¾ cup crushed pineapple, drained, juice reserved for the glaze

1 teaspoon almond extract

FOR THE GLAZE

1 cup confectioners' sugar

⅛ teaspoon ground cardamom

3 tablespoons reserved pineapple juice

½ teaspoon lime zest

½ cup unsweetened coconut chips

MORE TO SHARE RECIPE

NOTE

Unsweetened coconut flakes would also work as a great topping. Bonus points if you toast the coconut flakes!

1. **MAKE THE BREAD:** Preheat the oven to 350°F. Coat a 9 by 5-inch loaf pan with nonstick spray or butter.

2. In a medium bowl, whisk together the flour, baking powder, baking soda, and salt. Set aside.

3. In a large bowl, use an electric mixer on medium speed to beat the butter and both sugars until light and fluffy, about 2 minutes. At low speed, add the eggs, one at a time, beating well after each addition. Continue to beat until the mixture is smooth and fluffy, about 2 minutes.

4. Switching from the mixer to a large spoon, add the banana, pineapple, and almond extract and mix gently to combine. Slowly add the dry ingredients to the wet, mixing just until fully incorporated.

5. Pour the batter into the prepared pan, giving the pan a good shake to help the batter settle in evenly. Bake until a toothpick comes out clean when inserted into the center of the loaf, about 55 minutes.

6. Place the pan on a cooling rack and let cool for 10 to 15 minutes. Carefully loosen the bread from the sides of the pan. Invert the bread onto a cooling rack, then turn it upright and cool completely.

7. **MAKE THE GLAZE:** In a medium bowl, whisk together the confectioners' sugar and cardamom. Add the pineapple juice, 1 tablespoon at a time, mixing well after each addition. The consistency of the glaze should be a little thicker than heavy cream, pourable but not runny. Stir in the lime zest.

8. With the tines of a fork, gently pierce the top of the cooled bread, making small holes to absorb the glaze. Slowly pour the glaze over the loaf, using an offset spatula to spread it evenly over the top. Sprinkle coconut chips over the top.

Then the Lord said to Moses, Behold, I will rain bread from the heavens for you; and the people shall go out and gather a day's portion every day, that I may prove them, whether they will walk in My law or not.

EXODUS 16:4, AMPC

When God delivered the Israelites from slavery in Egypt, they were thankful, joyful, and relieved. But as they trudged through the wilderness, those feelings began to fade. Instead of keeping their eyes on the promised land, they began to see the hardships in front of them. They did not bring their anxiety, exhaustion, or fear to the Lord. Instead, they let it turn to grumbling, complaining, and restlessness.

It's easy to recognize God's goodness in the context of larger events. We praise him when we get the job we have been hoping for or when we celebrate a birth in the family. We profess his goodness when we experience healing or restoration in a relationship. God's goodness shows up daily, though, and not just in the favorable final outcomes. Sometimes we need to go back to discovering how to be grateful in the in-between moments, in simply waking up in the morning and thanking God for being able to take a breath.

Sometimes his goodness comes in the form of his favor, whether it's an opportunity you did not see coming or simply a friend dropping off a cup of coffee. It can be found in his protection or the gentle nudge we feel in our heart when we bring things to him in prayer. Or that gut feeling when we decide to say no.

To be honest, the thought of practicing gratitude in this manner used to frustrate me. That all changed when I faced a serious illness. Then I realized that the ability to wake up without a struggle was indeed something to be grateful for. Being able to navigate my days without physical hindrance or enduring symptoms or effects of treatment was a blessing. With so much going on in our lives at times, it can be easy to forget that our daily provisions are a result of his goodness in our lives. For the Israelites, the blessing and provision was something as small as manna.

> The people of Israel called the bread manna. It was white like coriander seed and tasted like wafers made with honey. Moses said, "This is what the LORD has commanded: 'Take an omer of manna and keep it for the generations to come, so they can see the bread I gave you to eat in the wilderness when I brought you out of Egypt.'"
>
> EXODUS 16:31–32

Even when they were ungrateful, God continually provided for the Israelites. Once the need had been met, they were on to whining about the next thing. We, too, forget that we have a God who sees us, who longs to provide not only for what we need but also for the desires of our heart. The simple fact is, we can come to him with our needs, and they will be met. Sometimes it's not exactly how we want or in what we consider the right timing. But when we see God's hand in our circumstances, it is always a sweet feeling.

———————

Dear Lord, thank you for waking me up each morning. Help me to slow down and see your goodness, no matter how big or small, in every day. I pray that I would bring my concerns and frustrations to you and that you'd give me the patience and wisdom I need to endure the waiting periods. Help me to listen carefully and discern your voice. Thank you for your protection and guidance.

No~Bake Cookie Butter Pie

SERVES: 8 | PREP: 20 MINUTES | INACTIVE: 2 HOURS 30 MINUTES

You have most likely come across a no-bake peanut butter pie, but have you ever been introduced to a cookie butter pie? If not, let me have the pleasure of introducing you to your newest obsession. Pile this high with fresh whipped cream and don't be surprised when half the pie is gone and you are the only one holding a spoon.

FOR THE CRUST

1 cup vanilla wafers

4 graham cracker sheets

¼ cup granulated sugar

½ teaspoon ground cinnamon

7 tablespoons unsalted butter, melted

FOR THE FILLING

¾ cup cookie butter

5 ounces cream cheese, softened

¾ cup confectioners' sugar

1 (8-ounce) container frozen whipped topping, thawed

1 recipe Quick Whip (page 216)

1. **MAKE THE CRUST:** In a food processor fitted with the S blade, process the vanilla wafers and graham crackers into fine crumbs. Transfer to a medium bowl. Add the sugar and cinnamon and mix to combine. Add the melted butter and stir until the mixture resembles wet sand.

2. Pour the crumb mixture into a 9-inch pie plate. Gently pat the crumbs over the bottom and up the sides of the plate to create a smooth, even surface. Do not pack the crumbs with too much force or else it will make the crust crack! Refrigerate until the crust is firm, about 30 minutes.

3. Meanwhile, **MAKE THE FILLING:** In a medium bowl, use a hand mixer on low speed to mix the cookie butter, cream cheese, and confectioners' sugar until smooth and fluffy, about 3 minutes.

4. Use a flexible spatula to fold in the whipped topping, mixing just until there are no white streaks of the topping. Pour the filling into the prepared crust and smooth the top with a spatula. Refrigerate until the filling sets, about 1 hour.

5. Spoon the Quick Whip over the top of the pie and spread over the surface. Return to the refrigerator for at least 1 hour before serving.

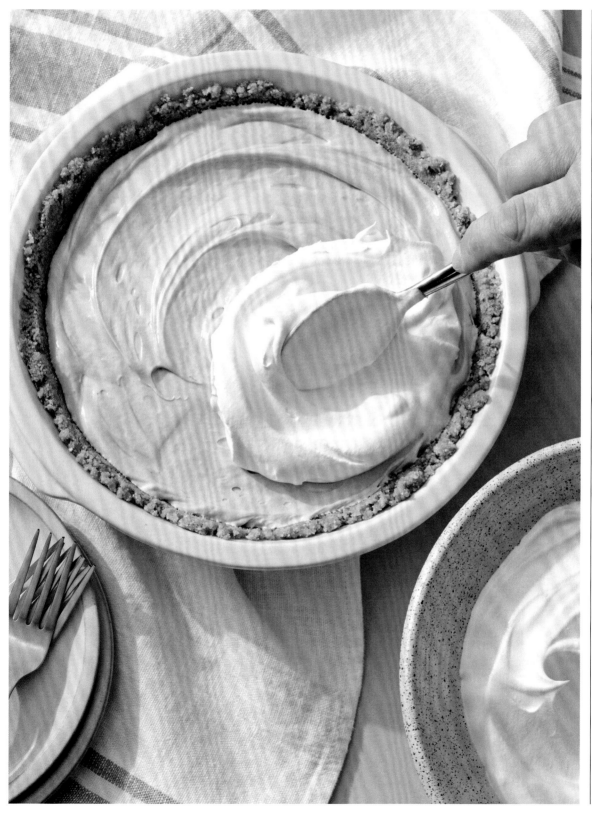

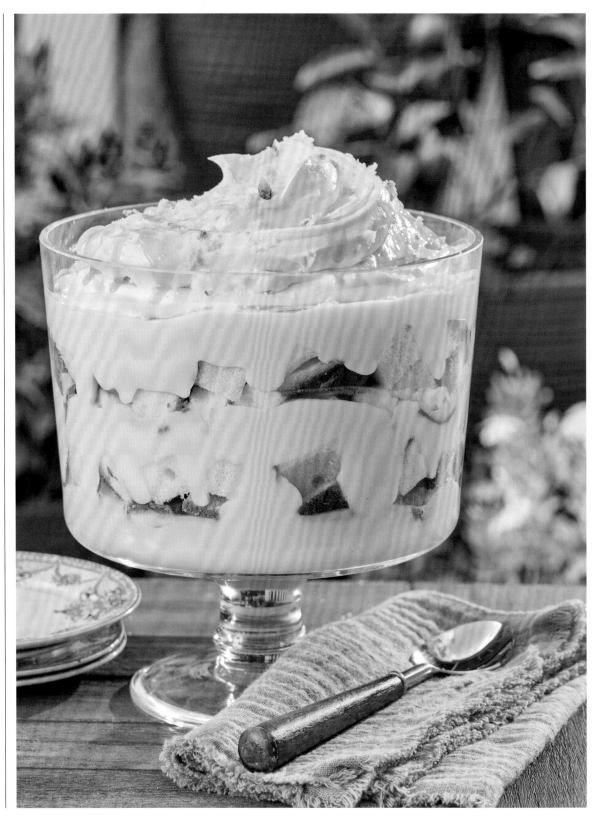

Toasted Almond Trifle

SERVES: 6 | PREP: 25 MINUTES | INACTIVE: 1 HOUR

A trifle is one of my favorite desserts for entertaining. While this trifle isn't fussy, it always proves to be a showpiece. Several different layers of cake, pudding, and fruit artfully arranged in a large glass bowl never seem to fail. It can be a mix of premade ingredients, or completely made from scratch—it doesn't matter.

½ cup amaretto liqueur

2 tablespoons granulated sugar

1 quart whole milk

2 (5.1-ounce) packages instant vanilla pudding

1 (8-ounce) container mascarpone cheese, room temperature

1 teaspoon almond extract

1½ cups well-chilled heavy cream

¼ cup confectioners' sugar

2 (11.5-ounce) pound cake loaves, cut into 1-inch cubes, plus 2 tablespoons of crumbs

1. In a small saucepan, boil the amaretto and sugar until the mixture thickens and is reduced by half, 3 to 4 minutes. Set aside to cool completely.

2. In a large bowl, whisk the milk and pudding mix to blend thoroughly, about 2 minutes. Set aside to thicken, about 5 minutes. Add the mascarpone and almond extract, whisking until smooth. Cover and refrigerate while you whip the cream.

3. In a large, chilled bowl, use a hand mixer to whip the cream, starting on low speed and gradually increasing to high, beating until soft peaks form, 2 to 3 minutes. Add the confectioners' sugar and continue beating until the cream thickens and the peaks become stiff enough to easily hold their shape.

4. To assemble the trifle, spread ½ cup of the pudding mixture evenly over the bottom of a trifle bowl or a clear glass bowl with straight sides such as a soufflé dish. Scatter 2 cups of the cubed pound cake over the pudding and top with 1 cup of the pudding. In this order continue layering: 2 cups of pound cake cubes, 1 cup of pudding, 2 cups of pound cake cubes, and 1 cup of pudding. Finish by spreading the whipped cream over the top. Drizzle with the amaretto syrup and sprinkle lightly with pound cake crumbs.

5. Cover and refrigerate for at least 1 hour, up to overnight, before serving.

Oatmeal Stuffed Apples

SERVES: 6 | PREP: 20 MINUTES | COOK: 45 MINUTES

Fun fact: Brian proposed to me in an apple orchard. Well, it was November, and all the apples were basically gone, but it's the thought that counts, right? No surprise, then, that apple desserts hold a special place in my heart. These stuffed apples are an even better version of a basic apple crisp. I love to use an apple liqueur from our favorite orchard, but apple brandy works just as well. This dessert will give your pumpkin pie some serious competition.

6 firm, crisp apples, such as Gala, Honeycrisp, or Jonagold

¾ cup rolled oats

¾ cup raisins

½ cup chopped pecans

½ cup packed dark brown sugar, plus more for sprinkling on top

½ teaspoon ground cinnamon

¼ teaspoon kosher salt

½ cup apple liqueur or apple brandy

6 tablespoons unsalted butter, cut in 1-tablespoon pats

½ cup dry white wine

1. Preheat the oven to 400°F.

2. Cut the top off the apples to expose the center core. Being careful not to break through the skin, use a melon baller to hollow out the apples, removing the core and flesh, leaving enough thickness so the shape of the apple remains intact. Put the apples in a shallow baking dish just large enough to hold them.

3. Coarsely chop enough of the reserved apple to measure ½ cup, discarding any seeds. Transfer the apples to a medium bowl.

4. Add the oats, raisins, pecans, brown sugar, cinnamon, and salt to the chopped apples and stir gently to combine. Pour the apple liqueur over it and stir until the mixture is uniformly moistened.

5. Fill each apple cavity with about ½ cup of the oat mixture. Place a pat of butter and a light sprinkle of brown sugar on top of each filled apple.

6. Pour the wine in the bottom of the baking dish. Cover the dish with aluminum foil and bake for 20 minutes. Remove the foil and continue baking until the apples are tender, about 25 minutes more.

7. To serve, place the apples on dessert plates and spoon some of the pan juices over the top.

NOTE

The apples are wonderful served with vanilla ice cream or a dollop of whipped cream on the side!

You can store leftovers for up to 4 days and reheat them at 350°F in a glass or ceramic baking dish.

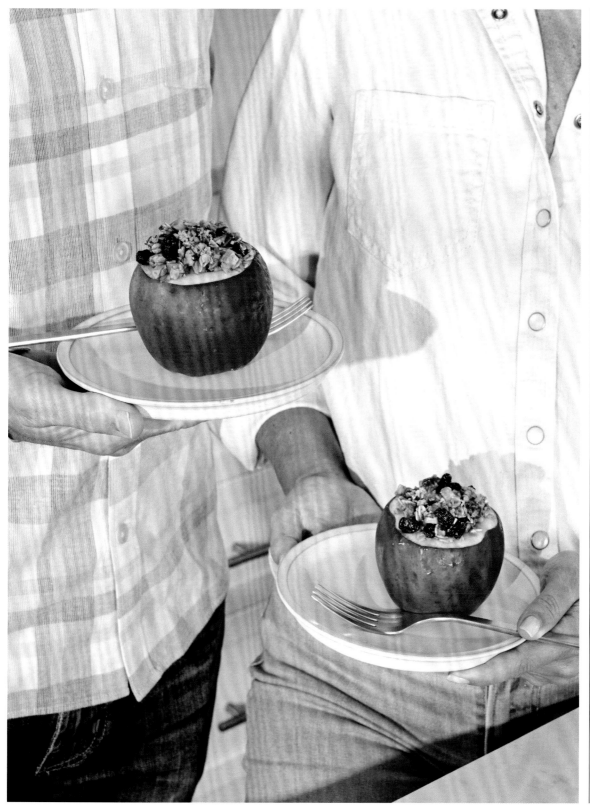

The LORD your God is with you,
   the Mighty Warrior who saves.
He will take great delight in you;
   in his love he will no longer rebuke you,
   but will rejoice over you with singing.

ZEPHANIAH 3:17

One of my greatest joys in this season of life has caught me off guard: watching Siena cheer for flag football. We had high hopes for her to become a soccer player, which she is. But she *loves* to cheer. She cartwheels incessantly, loves being a flyer for stunts, and beams with pride as she nails the halftime routine.

There is just something about watching her practice or standing in the rain at her games. It makes life busy and it takes up our Saturdays, but it has turned out to be good family time and something we look forward to each week. I love giving her a thumbs-up and smiling at her on the side-lines almost as much as I love seeing Brian grin and bear it as his dreams of his daughter playing soccer dance off into the sunset.

Do you ever imagine God almost as a cheerleader? I am not trying to be irreverent here or disrespectful, but I don't think he is as stuffy as some of us make him out to be. We know that he knows our number, so to speak. But as you make strides in your faith or overcome fear, can you imagine him cheering you on? As you finish a task he set before you, do you feel him running beside you, urging you to the finish line? Or maybe it is more of a Rocky situation. You have been knocked around a little, but he is refueling you, pouring water over your head, giving you a pep talk, and helping you reposition yourself for the next round.

In the Gospels, a blind man named Bartimaeus continually called out to Jesus for healing, despite others trying to quiet him down. Jesus heard him and stopped, and he asked the disciples to reach out to him. The disciples gave Bartimaeus a quick pep talk of sorts.

So they called to the blind man, "Cheer up! On your feet! He's calling you." Throwing his cloak aside, he jumped to his feet and came to Jesus.

MARK 10:49–50

Sometimes we forget that God is truly in our corner. When we seek him, call out to him, he always responds.

Do you know that we bring him joy just the same way our children and loved ones bring us joy? Not only is he coming alongside us, guiding us through the hard things and trudging through the trenches with us, he also is celebrating with us at the finish line. He is not just looking for our suffering. He wants to see us enjoy the life he has given us. It is very possible they know the "Cha-Cha Slide" in heaven.

Today, imagine God smiling with you, holding a big sign at the end of a finish line. Maybe his face is even painted in your colors. He wants to celebrate with you! It is easy to imagine him disappointed or upset with us. But make no mistake, he also wants to come alongside you and rejoice.

Dear Lord, help me know the depths of your love for me. Help me be reminded that you are my strength and my joy and that you want me to succeed according to your will. You died so that we could be free, so help me to tap into that freedom, rather than the bondage of sin. Help me see you as a good father, who urges me on to the finish line.

9

On~Hand Recipes

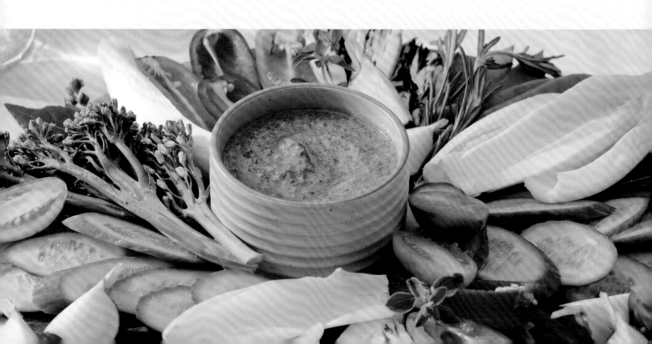

Having a great pesto, pickled vegetables, or a perfectly balanced salad dressing stocked in the fridge can take your everyday recipes to another level. It can also save money as they become staples. For example, having a great dressing recipe saves you from having to put one on your grocery list. It can also double as a great marinade.

Pickled onions can make a sandwich go from ordinary to mouthwatering. Stack them on top of burgers or even throw them in omelets. A good pesto can complement a veggie board or pasta dish any day. Flavored simple syrups can be used in coffees and cocktails and to liven up dessert dishes. The point is, these ingredients have the ability to make something feel a lot more special with very little effort!

Quick Pickled Red Onions

MAKES: 2 CUPS | PREP: 10 MINUTES | COOK: 5 MINUTES | INACTIVE: 30 MINUTES

I love having a batch of these quick pickled onions stashed in the fridge. I throw them on sandwiches and salads, and I also use them in bowls and as topping for tacos or nachos. The options are endless—the only thing I do not put them on is ice cream!

1 cup distilled white vinegar

½ cup red wine vinegar

1 tablespoon kosher salt

1½ teaspoons sugar

1 medium red onion, thinly sliced
  into half moons

2 garlic cloves, smashed

1 teaspoon whole black peppercorns

1 teaspoon whole mustard seeds

1 teaspoon dried dill

1. In a small saucepan, bring both vinegars, the salt, and sugar to a simmer, stirring to dissolve the sugar. Remove from the heat and cool completely.

2. Put the onions, garlic, peppercorns, mustard seeds, and dill in a 1-quart glass container. Add the pickling liquid, cover, and refrigerate for at least 2 hours or up to 2 weeks before using.

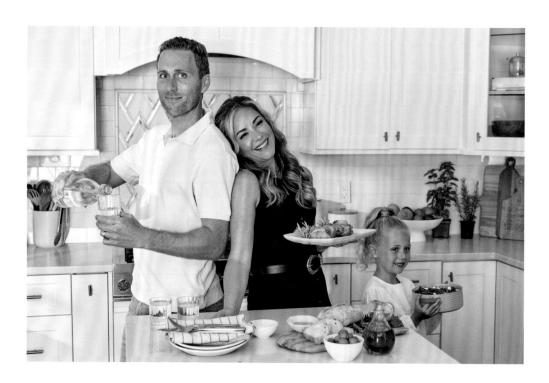

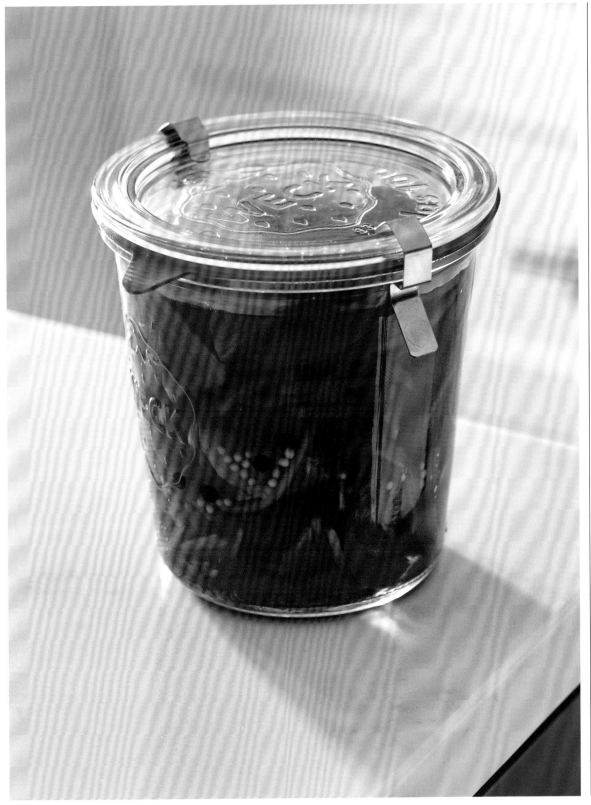

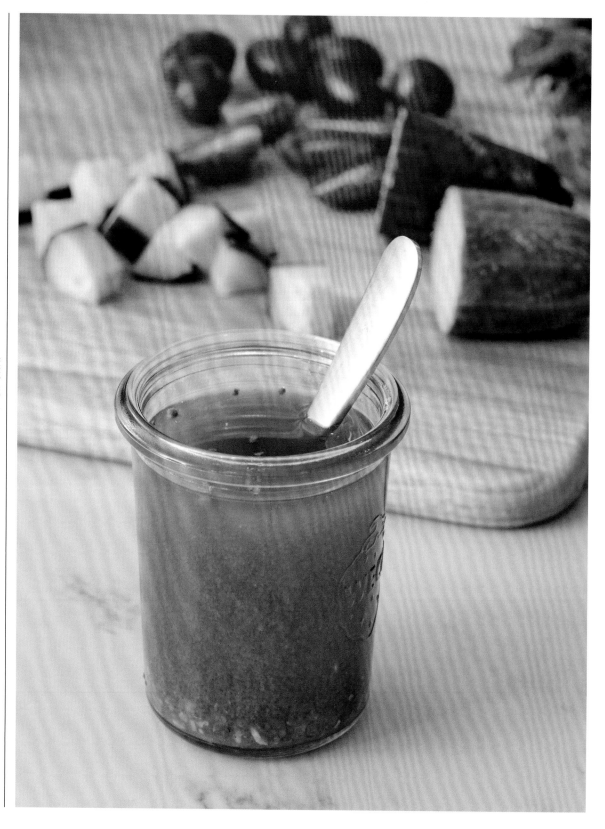

Everyday Dressing

I very rarely buy bottled dressing, mostly because I find myself making this particular dressing every other day. The only drawback is Siena will only eat salad with my dressing on it!

¼ cup extra-virgin olive oil

1 tablespoon red wine vinegar

1 teaspoon balsamic vinegar

1½ teaspoons minced garlic

¼ teaspoon Dijon mustard

¼ teaspoon dried oregano

¼ teaspoon kosher salt

⅛ teaspoon pepper

Pinch of granulated sugar

1. In a 1-cup liquid measuring cup, whisk together the oil, both vinegars, garlic, mustard, oregano, salt, pepper, and sugar. The dressing can be used immediately or refrigerated in an airtight container for up to 1 week.

Walnut Pesto

MAKES: 1 CUP | PREP: 10 MINUTES

This recipe uses walnuts instead of the pine nuts more traditionally called for. It also uses spinach, rather than just basil, in the mix, which gives it a little boost in the greens department! This pesto is great to have in your fridge for pasta dishes or as dip for a gorgeous veggie platter. I also find myself adding it to sandwiches or putting a dollop on top of homemade pizza!

1 cup packed fresh basil leaves

1 cup packed fresh baby spinach leaves

½ cup chopped walnuts

¼ cup freshly grated Parmesan cheese

3 garlic cloves, roughly chopped

2 tablespoons freshly squeezed lemon juice

¼ teaspoon crushed red pepper flakes

½ teaspoon kosher salt

⅛ teaspoon ground black pepper

½ cup extra-virgin olive oil

1. In a food processor fitted with the S blade, pulse the basil, spinach, walnuts, cheese, garlic, lemon juice, red pepper flakes, salt, and pepper to chop the ingredients.

2. With the machine running, add the oil in a steady stream and mix to a uniformly fine texture. The pesto can be used immediately or refrigerated for at least a week.

NOTE

For a pound of cooked pasta, about ½ cup of pesto is the right amount. As always, save some of the pasta cooking water to thin the sauce as needed.

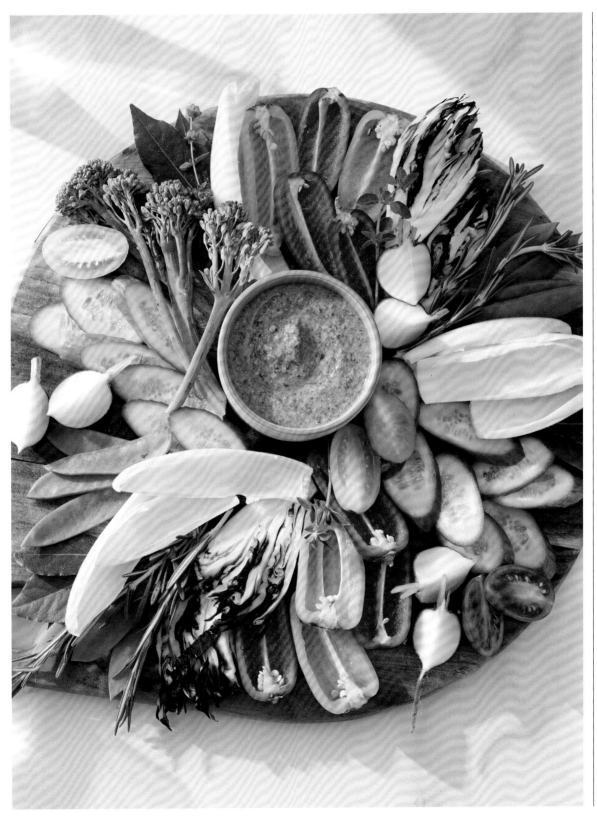

Quick Whip

MAKES: 2 CUPS | PREP: 5 MINUTES

You may be thinking, is this really worth it? Do I really want to make whipped cream from scratch? The answer is a resounding *yes!* Making whipped cream is so simple, yet it makes something feel so special. Even if you're just adding a dollop to a bowl of berries, it instantly impresses people. It also tastes so much better than anything you get out of a can!

1 cup heavy cream, well chilled

2 tablespoons confectioners' sugar

1 tablespoon vanilla extract

1. In a large bowl, using a hand mixer on low speed, begin to whip the cream. As it starts to form bubbles, gradually increase the speed to high and whip until the cream holds soft peaks. Add the sugar and vanilla and continue to beat until the peaks are somewhat stiff and firm, easily holding their shape. Toward the end, take care not to take it too far or small curds will form.

2. The whipped cream can be used immediately or refrigerated in a tightly covered container for up to 24 hours.

NOTE

Before making the whipped cream, put your stainless steel bowl in the fridge or freezer to make it cold. This will help the whipped cream come together quicker!

This is a great topping for No-Bake Cookie Butter Pie (page 200) and Spiced Chocolate Mousse (page 193).

Mint Simple Syrup

MAKES: 1 CUP | PREP: 5 MINUTES | COOK: 5 MINUTES | INACTIVE: 30 MINUTES

Simple syrups, both plain and flavored, are wonderfully versatile and not just for cocktails. In an instant, they can jazz up fruit salad, a bowl of oatmeal, and even your coffee and iced tea. I love how seemingly ordinary ingredients can yield extraordinary results.

1 cup sugar

3 sprigs fresh mint

1. In a small saucepan, bring 1 cup of cold water and the sugar to a boil over medium heat, stirring until the sugar has dissolved. Add the mint and reduce the heat to low. Simmer to thicken the syrup and infuse it with mint flavor, about 5 minutes.

2. Carefully remove and discard the mint. Cool the syrup and transfer to an airtight container. Refrigerate for up to 2 weeks.

Brown Sugar Simple Syrup

MAKES: 1 CUP | PREP: 5 MINUTES | COOK: 5 MINUTES | INACTIVE: 30 MINUTES

1 cup packed dark brown sugar

1. In a small saucepan over medium heat, bring 1 cup of cold water and the sugar to a boil, stirring until the sugar has dissolved. Reduce the heat to low and heat to a simmer. Cook until the syrup thickens slightly, about 5 minutes.

2. Cool the syrup, then transfer it to an airtight container and refrigerate for up to 2 weeks.

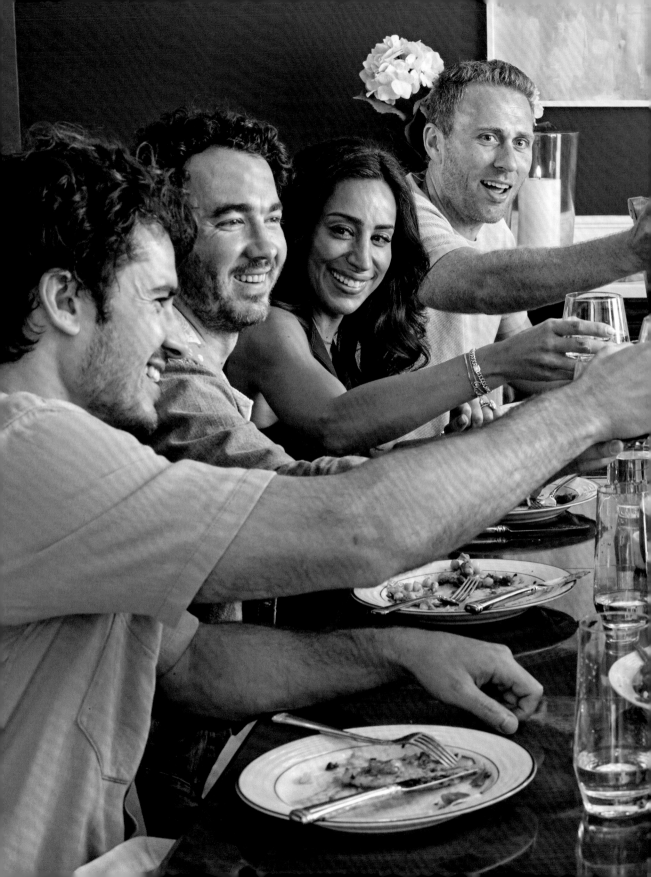

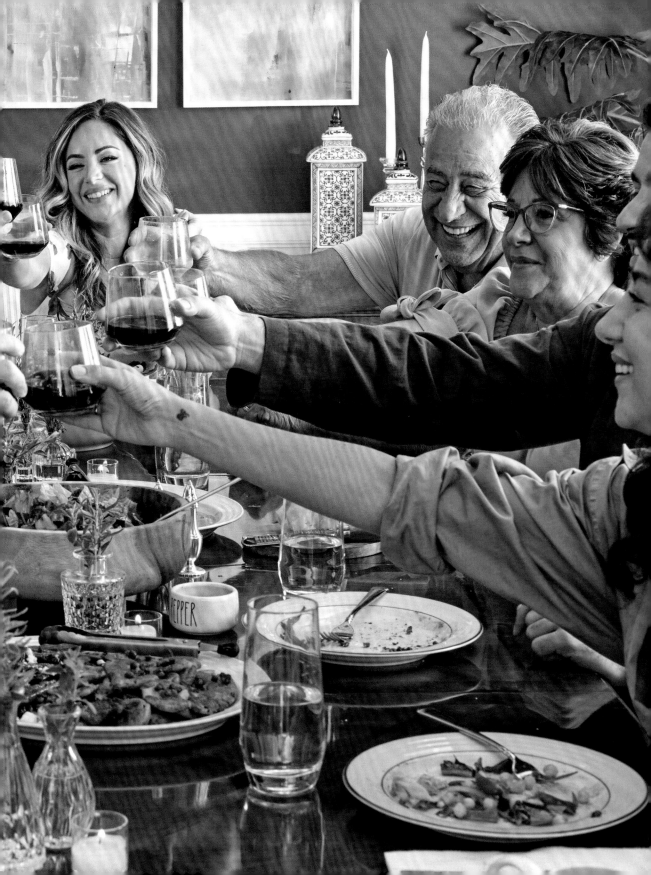

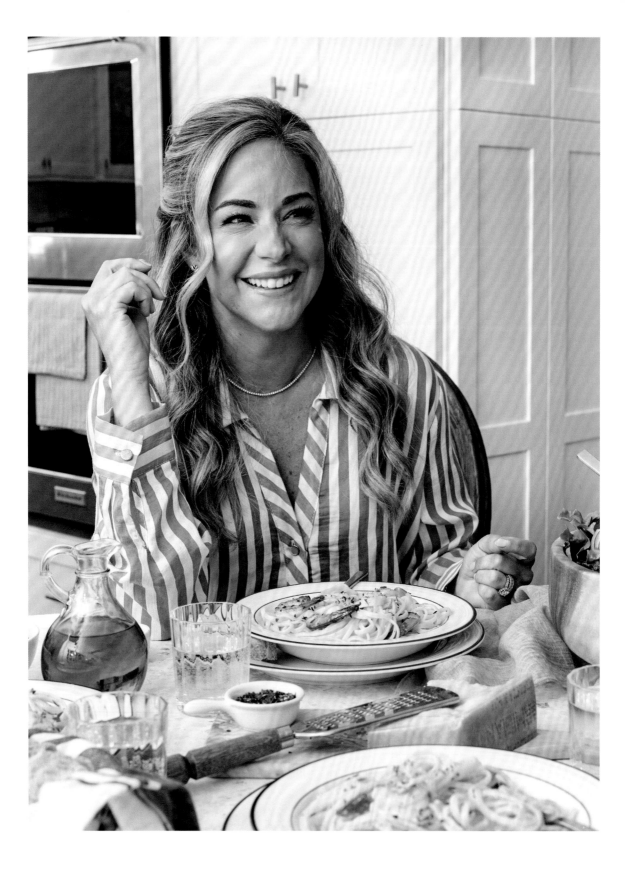

Acknowledgments

Thank you to those of you who have been following along with DishItGirl for more than ten years. Your consistent encouragement has been so valuable. You have cheered me on to this point. I hope this book encourages your heart and helps you make memories with those you love. I am overjoyed to finally give you a tangible piece of my heart!

A big thank you to Convergent and Penguin Random House for welcoming me into your family. I am so proud to be a part of a team with such heart! I know it takes many people to make a book come to fruition. From the marketing team to the copy editors and production, I am grateful for each one of you! I appreciate all the time and care that went into making sure this book was everything it has come to be.

To my church family, thank you for your consistent prayers from childhood until now. So many of you helped in forming my faith and encouraged me to continue seeking God's will for my life. You've come alongside my family in times when the valley has been present. And for the ladies who God has brought into my life more recently, thank you for encouraging me to keep leaning in to God's purpose in my life.

To my friends who are family, thank you for letting me cook for you in dorm rooms, my parents' house, and eventually my family home. From watching our parents have coffee together while we played to now doing it with our own children, we have grown together and I know it is a unique gift.

To Josie Sanchez, Ashley Schmidt, Grace Dutches, Jill Scarpa, Alyssa, and Tina Louise, thank you for helping me clean up my regular mess, haha! Josie and Tina, you made sure I broke out of my usual mom bun. Ashley, Grace, and Jill, thank you for giving this a girl a glow!

Kathleen Kerr, I am convinced my proposal sat on my computer for years waiting for our paths to cross. I am so grateful to Jill and Steph at Christian Parenting for being sensitive to that little nudge God gave them and introducing us. I am quite certain you are an answer to prayer. What a gift to have someone in your corner who understands your God-given assignment. Thank you for advocating for me as well as guiding me through this process—along with all my panicked and not-so-panicked text messages!

Derek Reed, thank you for pushing me beyond myself to be a more thoughtful writer. Helping me streamline my thoughts is *not* an easy task. You helped ensure that this book would speak into the lives of those who are meant to read it. Thank you for taking on this first-time writer with much patience and grace.

Dawn Miller and Carrie Parente, I could never say thank you enough for your talent and time. Watching both of you cook was probably the best learning experience. I was consistently blown away watching you make my food even better and more beautiful. You instantly felt like family, and my kitchen often feels empty without you!

Mike Krautter, what an honor to have you as part of this project. Thank you for lending not only your tremendous talent but also your heart. You didn't just take a photo and move on. I watched as you put great care and thought into each dish. Beyond that, you guided me through the shoot process with such patience. Thank you for helping this come to life in a way I couldn't have dreamed of!

Anthony Contrino, this book is just about as much yours as it is mine. Yes, you are a phenomenal food and prop stylist and a meticulous project manager! However, it is your heart that supersedes all of this. You did not need to essentially take me under your wing. You devoted time to teach me about recipe writing for real, answered every question, and were a sounding board to my constant questioning. You kept encouraging me as things became challenging along the way in a way we didn't foresee. This experience, as hard as it has been at times, was a dream because you were helping lead the way. You are not just a stylist or a project manager, but a true friend. It is going to be one of my greatest joys to wash dishes at your book shoot!

To my extended family, from those who are around the corner to those who are cities and states away, perhaps you see yourself in photos. You are part of the memories that live in my heart. These memories created comfort, joy, and peace at different times in my life. This helped inspire my desire to continue our traditions. Nina and Nicole, thank you for being the family I celebrate with not only in the book but throughout life, always.

Alena and Valentina, your "Ziti" loves you! One of my favorite memories will always be making you pancakes and raspberry oatmeal. I not so secretly love hearing your laughter and chaos behind me as I clean up at the kitchen sink. One of my reasons for having Sunday dinners and everything in between is seeing you together with Siena. Although the three of you will grow older, making you chicken cutlets never will!

To Danielle, Mikey, Katie, Kevin, and Nick—my OG and forever taste testers. Thank you for filling my table and life with so much pure joy. I am so proud of all your personal accomplishments, but above all else how you share in the commitment of keeping us together—that you take planes, trains, and whatever else to make it back to the table. Even if it sometimes must be gluten-free, carb-free, or whatever it is that month.

To my dad, the infamous "Bucky." My most treasured title is "You're Bucky's daughter." Thank you for taking me along to every bakery, deli, "hole in the wall," and everywhere in between. You're such a wonderful partner to Mom, as you've worked together to create the many memories we have at home. Thank you for always buying way too many pastries and "too much" antipasto. But most of all, thank you for making sure our meals never start without a prayer. For you know that is where the true legacy lies. Now my family and I have a gift that is everlasting.

To my mother, who dedicated her life to her family in every way possible and who served without knowing it was ministry. Your continued selflessness was the biggest lesson in motherhood I could have. Every dinner you put on the table during the week and beyond keeps us coming together even now. You created traditions that yielded lasting memories. You opened your home consistently in an effort to give us family and a sense of togetherness. And I say *effort* because I know now that it takes intentional effort. Your work was not wasted. Your table is now always full. Look at the pictures, look at this book—it is not just "my" work as you have stated, but it is inspired by you and happened because you worked with me.

Brian and Siena, you are the gift that God has given me, the family that I prayed for. I could not love you both more. Siena, you are the best little sous-chef and the food critic Mommy needs. Brian, we all know you totally won the lottery with me. However, one could say I am extremely blessed to have you by my side for this life. You will always be my favorite team to work with, and the people whom I love to cook for. Most of all, you're the ones I love building this life with.

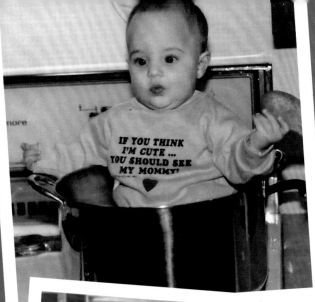

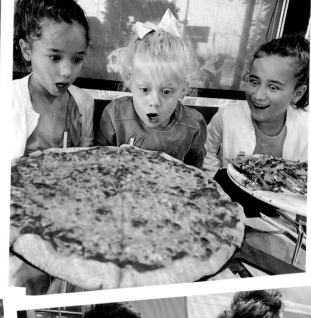

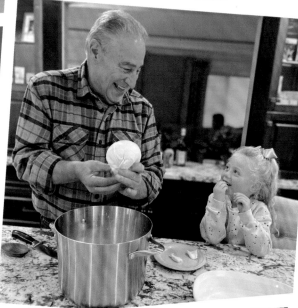

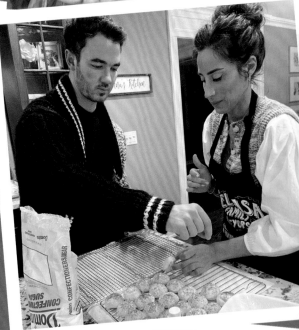

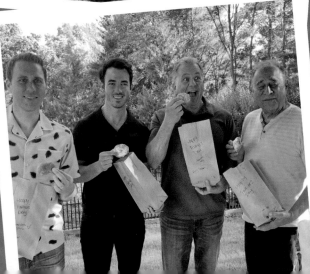

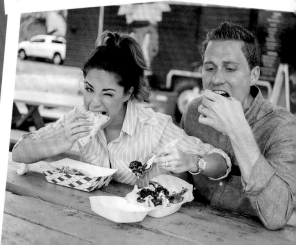

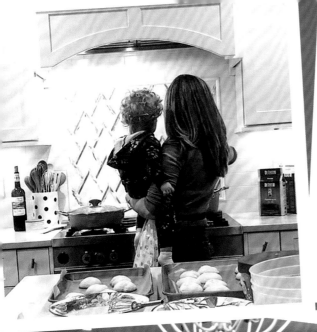
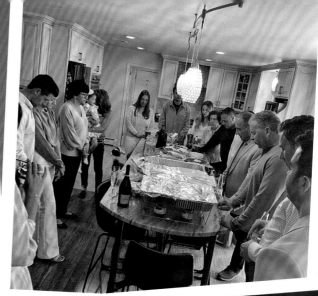
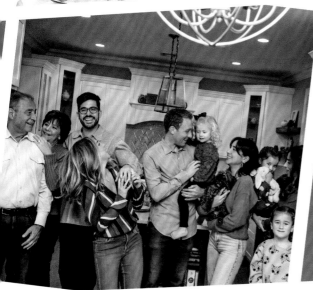
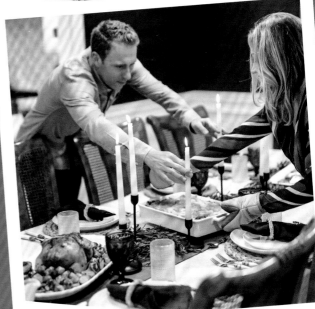
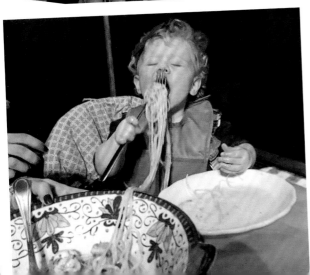
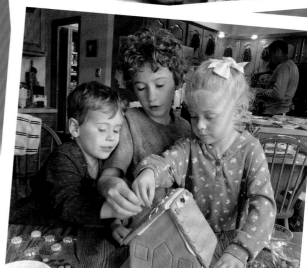

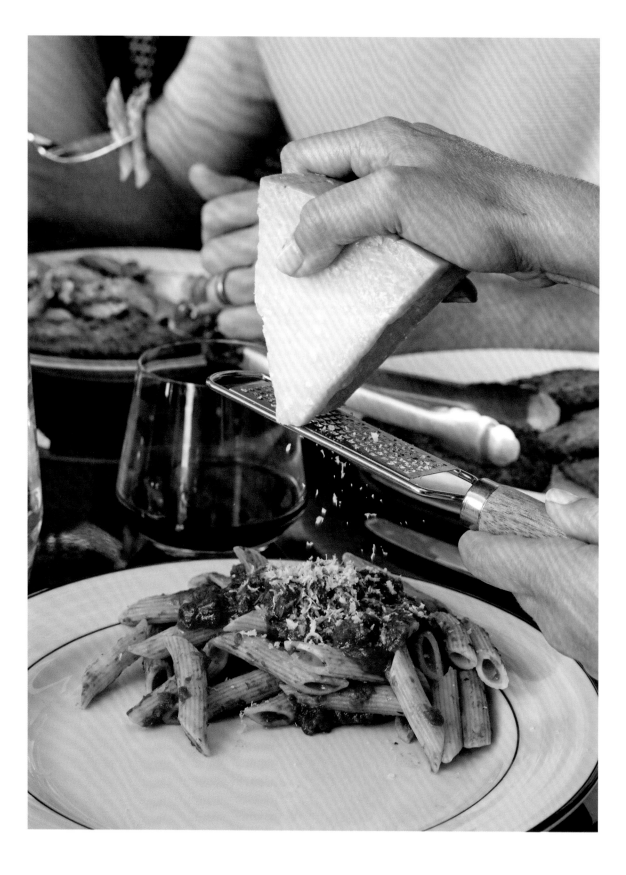

Index

INDEX

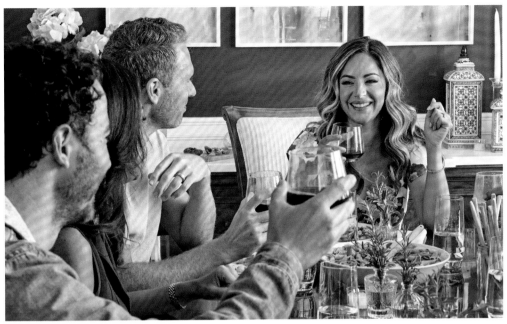

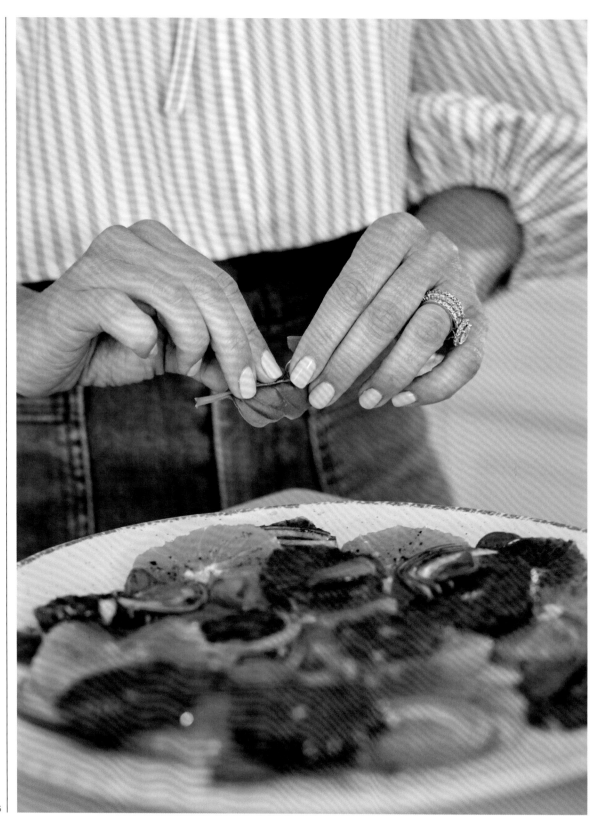

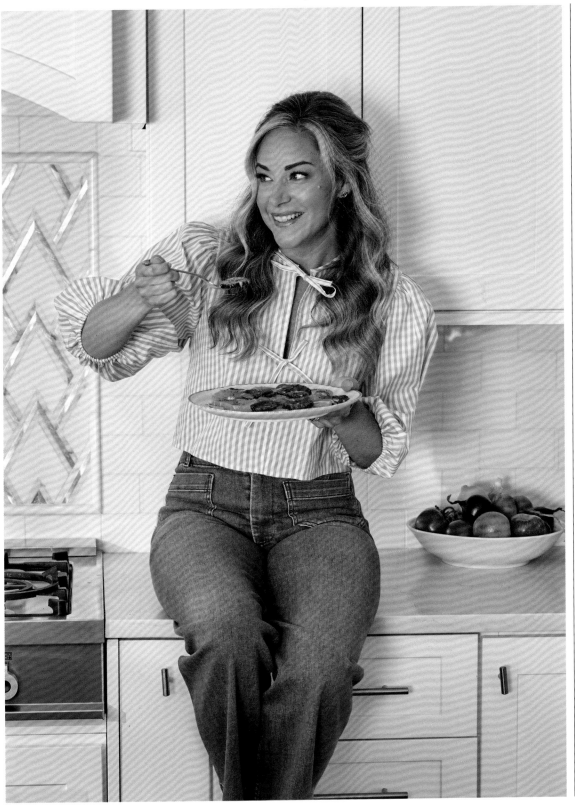

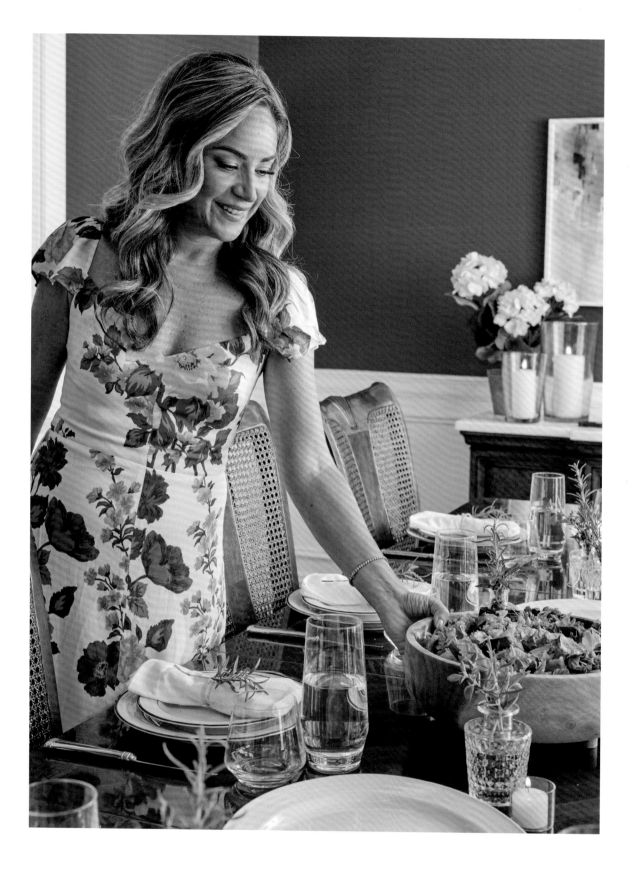

About the Author

DINA DELEASA-GONSAR is a recipe developer, author, speaker, and television personality behind the popular food blog DishItGirl.com. She is known for sharing her family traditions and modern twists on recipes, along with an inside look at her real life as a mom and wife. When in the kitchen, Dina brings her recipes to life with her personal anecdotes and honest, quick wit. Whether she's whipping up something quick for dinner or pulling out all the stops for a family celebration, she is inspiring at-home cooks to get creative and try dishes that will become catalysts for family gatherings that foster traditions.

Dina knows life isn't always glamorous, so she strives to keep her content relatable, making sure to dish out her real life that goes on behind the social posts and media platforms. Her family is at the center of everything she does. She can be seen sharing her recipes on national television and various media outlets. As a speaker and writer, she has lent her voice to the She Lives Fearless ministry as well as many other conferences and news outlets. It is part of Dina's mission to encourage other people to seek opportunities to gather with others and make memories, to help parents see that there is magnificence in what they consider mundane. She hopes to fill people with DishSpiration both in and out of the kitchen.

Whether it's a four-course meal or simply breakfast for dinner, with DishItGirl, Dina hopes to keep it real, with really good food along the way. She lives in New Jersey with her husband, Brian, and their daughter, Siena.

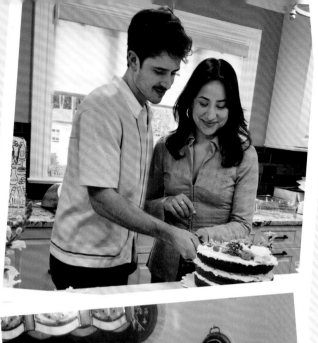
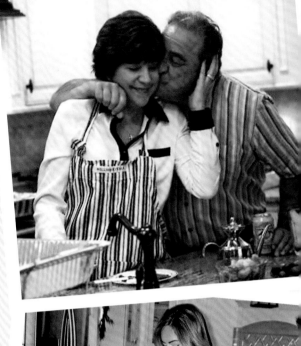
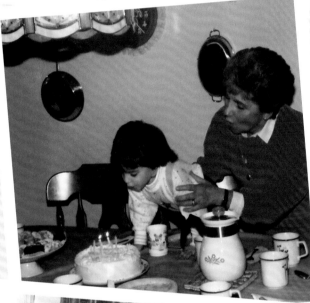
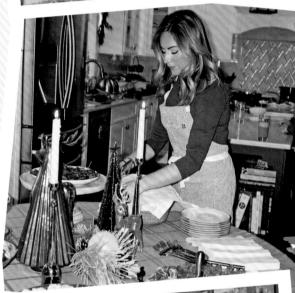
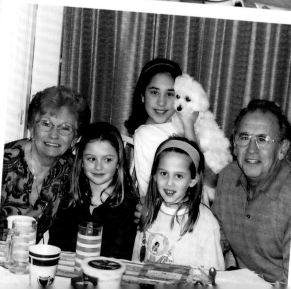
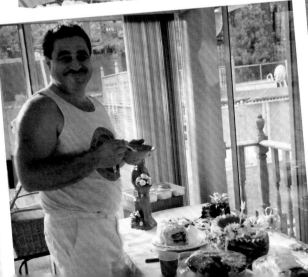

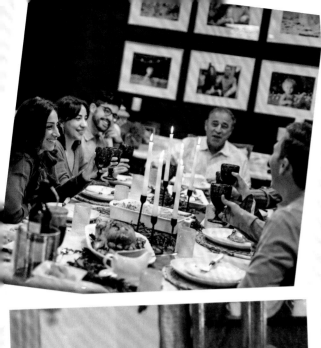
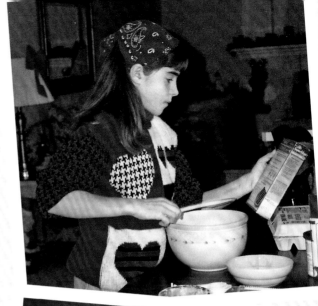
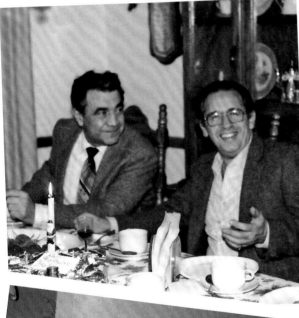
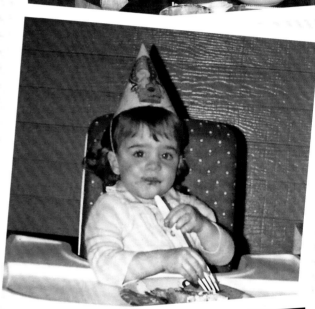
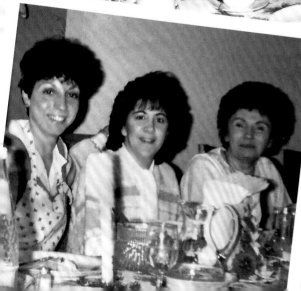
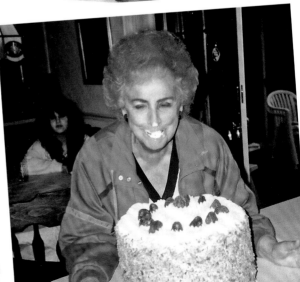

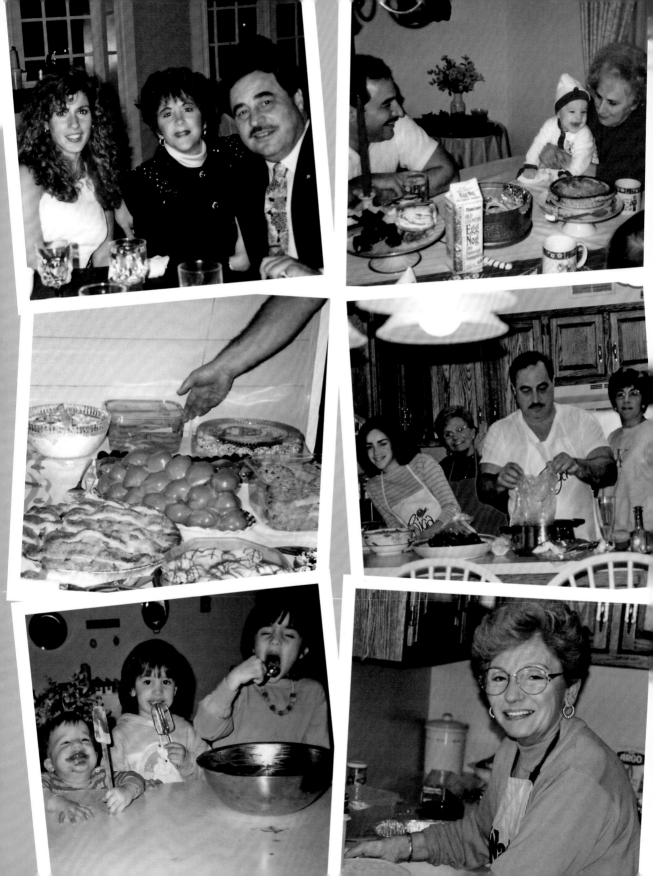